EPIDEMIOLOGY: AN INTRODUCTION

SOCIAL SCIENCE FOR NURSES AND THE CARING PROFESSIONS

Series Editor: Professor Pamela Abbott, Pro Vice Chancellor, Glasgow Caledonian University, Glasgow, Scotland

Current and forthcoming titles

EPIDEMIOLOGY:
AN INTRODUCTION

Graham Moon,
Myles Gould
and colleagues

OPEN UNIVERSITY PRESS
Buckingham • Philadelphia

Open University Press
Celtic Court
22 Ballmoor
Buckingham
MK18 1XW

email: enquiries@openup.co.uk
world wide web: http://www.openup.co.uk

and
325 Chestnut Street
Philadelphia, PA 19106, USA

First Published 2000

A catalogue record of this book is available from the British Library

ISBN 0 335 20012 5 (pbk)   0 335 20013 3 (hbk)

Library of Congress Cataloging-in-Publication Data
Epidemiology: an introduction / Graham Moon . . . [et al.].
    p.   cm. — (Social science for nurses and the caring professions)
    Includes bibliographical references and index.
    ISBN 0-335-20012-5 (pbk.) — ISBN 0-335-20013-3 (hc.)
    1. Epidemiology. I. Moon, Graham, 1956– II. Series.
    RA651 .E63 2000
    614.4—dc21
                                                          00-023300

Typeset by Graphicraft Limited, Hong Kong
Printed in Great Britain by Biddles Limited, Guildford and Kings Lynn

CONTENTS

SERIES EDITOR'S PREFACE

The health of populations is a major concern. Health Improvement Programmes and Health Action Zones are major initiatives to improve the health of the population. Epidemiology is a major tool for understanding the incidence and spread of disease in the population and therefore provides essential information for programmes such as these. Epidemiological research findings enable the development of policies and strategies to deal with the causes of diseases in the population. Research has, for example, established not only the links between cigarette smoking and lung cancer, and certain fats and heart disease but also the social class differentials in the incidence of these diseases.

An understanding of epidemiology and a knowledge of research findings is essential to underpin evidenced-based nursing practice. Nurses need to understand the incidence and spread of disease at population level and the causes in order to provide advice to patients and play their role in health promotion. This book will enable nurses to understand epidemiology, become aware of the major findings from epidemiological research and critically evaluate research papers. It will also provide a basic guide to those who wish to engage in epidemiological research. It complements the research methods text and reader in the series and the material on health inequalities in the social policy text.

Professor Pamela Abbott

PREFACE

This book is a collective effort. In putting it together we have drawn upon some fifteen years of experience in teaching epidemiology and epidemiological methods to health professionals and social scientists and providing epidemiological research services to health authorities. Over this period we have all worked together in various combinations and this collaborative approach has also guided the writing of the book. Chapters have each been authored initially by one or two individuals and then commented upon and revised within the group. Two of the authors (GM and MG) undertook the overall editing of the text. For the record, individual chapters were originated by the following individuals or pairs:

 1 Graham Moon
 2 Paul Iggulden and Myles Gould
 3 Paul Iggulden and Graham Moon
 4 Kelvyn Jones and SV Subramanian
 5 Kelvyn Jones and SV Subramanian
 6 Liz Twigg and Graham Moon
 7 Craig Duncan
 8 Myles Gould
 9 Tim Brown and Andrea Litva
10 Paul Iggulden and Myles Gould

All members of the authorial team are or have been associated with the Institute for the Geography of Health, University of Portsmouth.

Throughout the book we have endeavoured to simplify and summarize concepts within the text. Regular boxes elaborate on selected issues and offer activities designed to promote critical exploration. We recommend you read Chapter 1 carefully to gain a thorough grounding in the general concerns of epidemiological work. You may then choose to read Either Part 1 or Part 2, but a sequential approach, starting with Chapter 2 and following through to the end of the book, would be best. There is a series of activities at the end of each chapter. These are placed in this position to encourage you to revise each chapter as you go. While undertaking this revision we recommend you attempt each of the activities.

All web addresses provided were correct at the time the book went to press.

NOTES ON THE AUTHORS

Graham Moon is Professor of Health Services Research at the University of Portsmouth.

Myles Gould is Lecturer in Geography at the University of Leeds.

Kelvyn Jones is Professor of Geography at the University of Portsmouth.

Tim Brown, Craig Duncan and Liz Twigg are Research Fellows at the Institute for the Geography of Health, University of Portsmouth.

SV Subramanian is a research fellow at Harvard University.

Andrea Litva is Lecturer in Medical Sociology at the University of Liverpool.

Paul Iggulden is a project officer at the NHS Information Authority National Casemix Office.

ABBREVIATIONS USED IN THIS BOOK

AR	absolute risk
BHPS	British Household Panel Survey
CCCCP	Comprehensive Cardiovascular Community Control Programme
CDCP	Centers for Disease Control and Prevention
CDSC	Communicable Disease Surveillance Centre
CHD	coronary heart disease
DoH	Department of Health
EAR%	exposed attributable risk per cent
EBHC	evidence-based health care
ED	enumeration district
FCE	finished consultant episode
GHS	General Household Survey
GPRD	General Practice Research Database
GUM	genito-urinary medicine
HALS	Health and Lifestyle Survey
HRG	Healthcare Resource Group
HSE	Health Survey for England
ICD	International Classification of Disease
IHD	ischaemic heart disease
LBS	local base statistics
LS	Longitudinal Survey
MSGP	Morbidity Statistics from General Practice
NHS	National Health Service
NHSE	National Health Service Executive
NNT	number needed to treat
NRT	nicotine replacement therapy
ONS	Office for National Statistics
OPCS	Office of Population Censuses and Surveys
OR	odds ratio
PAR	pure attributable risk
PAR%	population attributable risk per cent
PHCDS	Public Health Common Data Set
PHLS	Public Health Laboratory Service
RAWP	Resource Allocations Working Party
RCGP	Royal College of General Practitioners
RCT	randomized clinical trial
RHA	regional health authority
RR	relative risk
SAR	Sample of Anonymised Records
SAS	small area statistics
SCPR	Social and Community Planning Research

SMR	standardized mortality ratio
SSRU	Social Statistics Research Unit
STD	sexually transmitted disease
UPA	underprivileged area
WHO	World Health Organization

WHAT IS EPIDEMIOLOGY?

Epidemiology has been defined as the study of patterns of disease occurrence in human populations and the factors that influence these patterns (Lilienfeld and Lilienfeld 1980). It describes, quantifies and postulates causal mechanisms for health phenomena in the population. This involves the study of variations in levels of mortality (death) and morbidity (illness) between population groups and the testing of hypotheses concerning the reasons for such variations. It extends to the evaluation of the relative effectiveness of different approaches to treating disease. Box 1.1 exemplifies some typical findings from epidemiological research.

The main aim of this introductory chapter is to outline the distinctive character of the epidemiological approach to the analysis of health and disease. We also outline a range of purposes to which the epidemiological approach has been applied. There are three sections to the chapter:

- An exploration of the key general characteristics of the epidemiological approach. This section examines such issues as the population focus of epidemiology, its concern with disease and its stress on quantitative methods of analysis.
- A consideration of the current areas in which epidemiology is applied. Here the intention is to give a flavour of what has been achieved by using the epidemiological approach.
- A concluding section that sets out the structure of the book and how it should be used.

Box 1.1 The epidemiology of tobacco smoking

Epidemiological research methodology suggests that smoking is a significant cause of excess mortality and morbidity:

- Current cigarette smokers in comparison with non-smokers have an overall 70 per cent excess mortality regardless of amount of smoking.
- Mortality from smoking increases with the quantity of cigarettes smoked, the duration of smoking, starting at earlier ages, and amount of smoke inhaled.
- Associations have been observed between smoking and morbidity from cardiovascular diseases; cancer of the lung, larynx, mouth, bladder and pancreas; non-neoplastic bronchopulmonary diseases; and peptic ulcer disease.
- The ill effects of smoking are made worse by occupational exposures to asbestos, chromium, nickel and other potentially toxic or carcinogenic materials.
- Smoking is a direct cause of reduction in birth weight and increased prenatal mortality.
- Cessation of smoking can eliminate or greatly reduce the health threat.

Epidemiology defined

Put simply, epidemiology is concerned with the distribution and determinants of health and diseases, morbidity, injuries, disability and mortality in populations. It is about the health experiences of human communities. This focus involves rather more than simple set of facts or findings such as those set out in Box 1.1. Importantly it entails deployment of what Ashton (1994) has called the epidemiological imagination. This is a particular way of working and thinking about disease and illness which is quite distinct from that which has often prevailed in health care professional practice. This imagination is characterized by four major features: a focus on human populations; quantitative analysis of collected information; a strong practical, applied intent; and a high level of interdisciplinarity. An assessment of each of these features provides the organizing framework for the remainder of this section.

Population medicine

Epidemiology examines the distribution and determinants of disease occurrence among *population groups* rather than among individuals. Indeed, epidemiology is often referred to as 'population medicine'. While the starting point for this concern may be the impact of disease on individuals, the focus of analytical attention is firmly on the groups to which individuals belong. To illustrate this point, consider the following statement: 'the four patients were previously healthy homosexual men in their early 30s who resided in Los Angeles and first became ill in the 9 months ending in June 1981'. There are four epidemiological grouping factors evident in this sentence: health status (previously healthy); sociodemographic status (sexual orientation, sex, age); place (where the patients lived); and time (when the patients first became ill). It is these features that are traditionally used to characterize patterns of disease occurrence in epidemiological studies.

Any disease can be looked at in terms of the characteristics of the population groups getting that disease. The population perspective becomes interesting only when consideration is given to the relationship between the population groups and the distribution and determinants of a disease in question. In particular, epidemiologists will seek to discover whether the *distribution* of disease occurrence varies from one population group to another. For example, hypertension may be more common among young African American men than among young white men. Mortality from coronary heart disease may vary between Hispanics and non-Hispanics. An important principle of epidemiology is that human disease does not occur randomly. Diseases may have different distributions depending upon the underlying characteristics of the populations being studied.

Moving from disease distribution to **disease determinants** is the next logical step. Determinants are factors or events that are capable of bringing about a change in health. Some examples are specific biological agents that are associated with infectious diseases or chemical agents that may act as carcinogens. Other potential determinants may include less specific factors, such as stress or adverse lifestyle patterns (lack of exercise or a diet high in saturated fats). For the epidemiologist, a key question is the extent to which a group membership is linked to a disease determinant. Attention focuses on asking why certain diseases concentrate among particular population groups. This task is far from straightforward, either sociologically or methodologically. These difficulties are considered in greater depth in later chapters. At this stage it is perhaps sufficient to state that another important principle of epidemiology is that human disease has causal and preventive factors that can be identified via systematic investigation of who gets ill.

Thinking about the population distribution and determinants of disease also begs a further question: what is a disease? Although epidemiology may make much of its concern with populations and, as will be seen later in this chapter, this concern stands in possible contrast to the more traditionally individualist concerns of clinical medicine, epidemiology is generally reliant upon standard clinical definitions of disease. For example, it is important to be clear about the definition of coronary heart disease. The definitional process is aided by the existence of established international standards of diagnostic coding such as the **International Classification of Disease** (ICD), now in its tenth revision.

The language of quantification

Epidemiology makes extensive use of quantitative data. Its discussions of disease distribution and disease determination involve counting cases of disease and relating such data to other indicators. In short, epidemiological research is empirical and requires quantification of relevant factors.

Epidemiologists enumerate cases of disease to objectify subjective impressions concerning disease, such as a doctor's observations about the types of people among whom a disease seems to be common. Quantification also enables **standardization** according to demographic variables such as age, sex and race. This facilitates comparison between different datasets. Thirdly, a quantitative approach provides a basis for analysis. It enables the epidemiologist to employ statistical techniques or display tools such as graphs and tables that illustrate pictorially the frequency of disease.

Box 1.2 summarizes the characteristics of 941 confirmed cases of toxic shock syndrome that were reported to the US Centers for Disease Control and Prevention between 1970 and 1980 (CDCP 1981). It shows clearly how epidemiologists use quantified information. Note the italicized terminology; this is basic to epidemiology and will be encountered again and again throughout this book. Three further terms are also worthy of brief preliminary note:

Box 1.2 Toxic shock syndrome

The age range for female patients was 6–61 years, with a mean of 23 years. One-third of all cases occurred in women 15–19 years old. The age range for male patients was 6–58 years, with a mean of 23 years. Seven cases occurred in blacks, 3 in Asians, 3 in Hispanics, and 2 in American Indians. Seventy-three cases resulted in death (case fatality ratio = 7.8%).

(CDCP 1981)

We are given the range (aged 6 to 61), an overall summary measure of the average age of attack (a mean of 23 years), absolute counts of the number of occurrences by subgroups (e.g. 7 cases in blacks), a ratio of the dead to the living (a case fatality of 7.8%), and a relative frequency (one-third of all female deaths were in the 15–19 age group). The reason why epidemiology is so quantitative is that it is seeking *patterns* (in this case in terms of ethnicity, age and sex), and noting the inherent *uncertainty* involved in dealing with people and populations (not all 15–19 females report toxic shock syndrome, and while some people die from it, the overwhelming majority do not). An epidemiological study would go on to investigate, statistically, the relationship between this *outcome* (toxic shock syndrome) and *exposure* to potential causal or risk factors. The interest in uncertainty would be extended by considering the degree of confidence which could be placed in any such estimates of relationships.

● *Pattern*: who gets the disease; who gets successfully cured.
● *Uncertainty*: the degree to which the expected does not happen.
● *Outcome*: get the disease (or not); recover (or not).
● *Exposure*: experience the factor which is meant to lead to the disease.

- **Prevalence**: the number of *existing* cases of a disease or health condition in a specific population at some designated time or during some designated time period.
- **Incidence**: the number of *new* cases that come into being in a specified population during a specified period of time.
- *Risk*: the proportion of individuals who, on average, contract a disease of interest over a specified period of time. Risk is estimated by observing a particular population for a defined period of time – the *risk period*.

Practicality and applicability

The preceding sections hint at the uses of epidemiology. Epidemiology is concerned with efforts to describe, explain, predict and control. These aims have strong practical and applied relevance. *Description* means identifying cases of diseases in order to calculate the relative frequencies of the diseases within population subgroups. It can also mean discovering trends in the occurrence of diseases. *Explanation* entails discovering causal factors and, in the case of infectious diseases, modes of transmission. *Prediction* allows the estimation of the likely number of cases that will develop in the future. *Control* means applying epidemiological knowledge to prevent the occurrence of new cases of disease, eradicate existing cases, and prolong the lives of people with disease.

Taken together, these four aims can lead to an improved understanding of the natural history of disease (how diseases develop over time) and the factors that relate to disease distributions. With the knowledge that is obtained from such efforts, attention can proceed to intervention to reduce the impact of disease. In practical terms this applicability is likely to entail both descriptive work in which the focus is on patterns of disease in populations and more analytical studies where interest centres on the aetiology of disease (causes). Descriptive work might seek to distinguish groups with abnormal levels of disease. Aetiological research is concerned with the determinants of disease onset, with true cause-and-effect relations. If these are found it may be possible to develop better strategies for disease prevention.

Selective prevention targets those at high risk. In epidemiological terms this requires the ability to screen into separate high and low risk groups. The prevention has to be valid and effective with those at high risk. In contrast, **population-based prevention** is aimed at everybody and is concerned with reducing overall levels of risk. Resources are directed at the entire community with the aim of lowering disease levels for all, not just those most at risk. Having designed an intervention on the basis of epidemiological evidence, it is important then to provide *evaluation* of the intervention's effectiveness. This requires research to identify the important determinants of the diseases in question. In the past, many medical interventions were not subject to rigorous evaluation in terms of their effectiveness. The randomized clinical trial (RCT), a classic epidemiological technique, is now seen as the most rigorous method available for evaluating the effectiveness of an intervention.

Interdisciplinarity

Epidemiology is an area of study that is intensely interdisciplinary. It draws from statistical science and the social and behavioural sciences as well as from the biosciences and clinical medicine. This makes it an extraordinarily rich and complex science. Epidemiology profits from the interdisciplinary approach because the causality of a particular disease in a population may not be understandable from within the perspectives of just one discipline. *Statistical science* provides the underlying technical apparatus of much epidemiological research. It is critical to the evaluation of epidemiological data and particularly to the measurement of risk and uncertainty. The *social sciences* elucidate the role of race, social class, education, cultural group membership and behavioural practices in health-related phenomena. Furthermore, much of the methodology of sampling, measurement, questionnaire development, design and delivery, and methods of group comparison are borrowed from the social sciences. *Microbiology* may provide information about specific disease agents, including their morphology and modes of transmission, while *toxicology* can help to identify the presence and health effects of chemical agents, particularly those found in the environment and the workplace. *Clinical medicine* is involved in the diagnosis of the patient's state of health, that is, defining whether the patient has (or had) a particular disease or condition.

Types of epidemiology

Epidemiological researchers are increasingly realizing that the causes of ill health may operate at a number of different levels: *internally*, within the body; *behaviourally*, at the level of an individual; and *contextually* and *structurally*. These levels are related. Heart disease may reflect cholesterol levels (internal), dietary decisions (behavioural), or poverty (structural). A useful analogy that makes this point is that of 'focusing upstream'. While the immediate causes of disease may indeed be internal to the body, these internal causes may reflect behavioural factors, themselves constrained by structure. It is now common to recognize different types of epidemiology which differ in the stress they place on these understandings of disease causation.

Clinical epidemiology studies the individual patients; aetiological studies focus on the internal mechanics of the body. Medical journals, such as the *British Medical Journal*, are excellent sources of examples of such work. Studies will normally involve clinically based measurements of the biochemical or physical functioning of samples individuals. Among many classic studies of the clinical variety is Morris (Chair) (1968). This was a dietary study of older men recovering from a heart attack and involved comparison of different dietary regimes with measured content of saturated fat against outcome measures of serum cholesterol levels. The study revealed a significant fall in serum cholesterol for those with diets with low levels of saturated fats and was instrumental in setting recommendations for 'healthy' post-heart-attack diets.

Social epidemiology considers determinants of health and illness that are rooted in the divisions of contemporary society. The determinants are not single agents such as specific bacteria or other biological determinants of disease. Nor are they necessarily merely demographic variables, such as age or sex. Rather, they are concerned with the influence of a person's position in the social structure upon the development of disease (class, location, employment status and so on) and with the impact of behavioural factors. Historically, much epidemiology took this form and today the health inequalities literature covers much common ground. Among the most significant studies are those of Sir Richard Doll and colleagues linking smoking to lung cancer (Doll and Hill 1964; Doll and Peto 1981).

Critical epidemiology places an emphasis on the social and power relations that shape disease definition and disease causation. This approach uses qualitative as well as quantitative methodologies. There is a concern for causation and prevention but action is seen to be required at the population level. We look in greater detail at this somewhat different perspective in Chapter 9.

More generally, epidemiology can also be distinguished by the type of disease it is studying, the 'environment' in which it is practised, and the knowledge that it regards as legitimate. Thus, under the first heading, **communicable-disease epidemiology** focuses on diseases that can be spread or 'caught'. Such diseases are less common than they once were in the western world but communicable disease epidemiology retains an importance in the developing world and has continued relevance to the West in the study of AIDS/HIV and resurgent tuberculosis. **Chronic-disease epidemiology** considers conditions such as heart disease and cancers that are overwhelmingly the major killers in western society and are now seen to involve behavioural and contextual factors.

The environment in which epidemiology is practised is a distinguishing factor for **community epidemiology** in which a stress is placed on disease surveillance and occurrence in real-world settings, screening and the implementation of community-based interventions. The classic work of John Snow on cholera in mid-nineteenth century London exemplifies this work (Snow [1855] 1936). **Occupational epidemiology** focuses on the workplace, monitors the levels of disease in the workforce, and looks for causal relations between occupational exposures and subsequent disease.

The legitimacy of a knowledge base underpins the realization that quantitative epidemiology is the underlying approach of **evidence-based medicine** in which interventions are subject to extensive critical appraisal and review so that only the most effective procedures are used in disease management. In contrast, **popular** or **lay epidemiology** sees experts like doctors, or even epidemiologists, removed from the frame of analysis and attention focused on accounts of disease causation which emphasize the qualitative views, opinions and knowledge of 'ordinary' people. For critics this can be anecdotal, uninformed or even dangerous. On a more positive note, and recognizing that most disease is self-treated, ignored or undiagnosed (the so-called **clinical iceberg**), popular epidemiology offers insight into the way in which most disease is most commonly understood and treated.

This book

This book is intended to provide a practical yet critically informed review of epidemiology. We consider epidemiology both as a toolkit of research methods for the study of disease and as an approach to understanding disease distributions. The structure of the book reflects these broad aims and is divided into two parts.

The next five chapters are concerned with how epidemiological studies are put together. We begin in Chapter 2 with a consideration of sources of data for epidemiological studies. These are reviewed and their quality is assessed. Chapter 3 then looks at general descriptive studies of disease frequencies and patterns using the example of coronary heart disease. This important chapter serves as a taster for the more analytical approaches covered in Chapters 4 and 5. It shows the initial importance of descriptive work in epidemiology. Chapter 4 considers the principles of analytic designs and exemplifies those principles with an assessment of the so-called gold standard of the randomized clinical trial experimental design. Chapter 5 examines observational studies and reflects upon choices in epidemiological research designs. The final chapter in Part 1 – Chapter 6 – sets out the basic techniques used for drawing quantitative conclusions from epidemiological research designs.

The second part of the book is simultaneously both more reflective and more practical. It contains four chapters. Chapter 7 looks back over the epidemiological designs presented in Part 1, draws together the themes they have raised and introduces a note of critique. This critical orientation is continued in Chapter 9 where we present an overtly sociological assessment of epidemiology as a generally conservative science in which people are reduced to objects of study. Chapters 8 and 10 step back from this possibly rather negative assessment and look at the way in which epidemiology is currently employed in the UK National Health Service (NHS). Chapter 8 considers the role of epidemiological studies in the development of an evidence-based health service while Chapter 10 reflects upon the day-to-day practice of epidemiology in NHS settings.

Summary

- Epidemiology is concerned with the distribution and determinants of health and diseases, morbidity, injuries, disability and mortality in populations.

- Epidemiology examines the distribution and determinants of disease occurrence among population groups rather than among individuals.

- Attention focuses on asking why certain diseases concentrate among particular population groups and on applying epidemiological knowledge to prevent the occurrence of new cases of disease, eradicate existing cases, and prolong the lives of people with disease.

- Much but not all epidemiological work uses quantitative methods and statistical analysis.

- It is possible to distinguish several different types of epidemiology.

Further reading

Ashton, J. (1994) *The Epidemiological Imagination*. Buckingham: Open University Press.

Activities

1 Choose an outcome of relevance to your interests as a health professional. Make a list of the exposures that you think might be worth investigating. By each exposure, write down the reasons why you think it is relevant.

2 Morris (1975) identified seven specific 'uses' of epidemiology:

   (a) *Historical*: recording changes in disease frequency over time.
   (b) *Community diagnosis*: identifying the size and nature of community health problems and the extent of health inequalities between groups.
   (c) *Risk assessment*: calculating the likelihood or risk of disease among population groups.
   (d) *Operational research*: do all groups benefit equally from same treatment?
   (e) *Completing the clinical picture*: improving understanding of the socio-demographic impact of disease.
   (f) *Identification of syndromes*: revealing connections or differences between conditions.
   (g) *Clues to causes*: making comparisons to highlight environmental/social factors which may underpin disease causation.

   To what extent do these 'uses' equate with areas of concern in your own professional environment? Try to rephrase these points into a series of potential epidemiological research questions relevant to your own area of interest.

3 Consider these two statements:

   'Disease is a matter for doctors. They test and diagnose individuals to identify the disease. Drugs and surgery provide the solution to health problems. Future advances will come from laboratory science enabling the development of better drugs and deeper knowledge about the workings of the human body.'

   'Only by combating social inequality can we really combat ill health. Social inequality lies at the root of disease and underpins what some have called the negative results of ignorance and health-damaging behaviour.'

Working with a colleague or a group of colleagues, use these two statements as the basis for a debate. At the end of your debate, evaluate the two statements critically for what they suggest about different types of epidemiology.

of a birth or death. In both cases, a data collection form is needed and the principles governing the design of these forms are fairly universal.

There are numerous texts on survey methods and it is not our purpose here to provide an exhaustive guide to how to do surveys. Interested readers should consult a classic specialist textbook such as Moser and Kalton (1971) or Hoinville *et al.* (1977). The key points to bear in mind, either when conducting your own survey, or when evaluating someone else's – or even when thinking about the ways in which **routine statistics** are originated – are:

● *Concept clarity*: are concepts explained clearly at the data collection stage and is there a shared understanding of what they mean? This might involve the wording of questions and the development of protocols to ensure that there are clear definitions of concepts.
● *Sampling*: while routine data should clearly cover users of services and those events where registration is required, other sources, with the exception of the national census of the population, will necessitate the sampling of some fraction of the population. This approach reflects practicality as well as a recognition that you seldom need to ask something of everyone before you have a good idea what the pattern of responses will be. The sampling method of choice is **random sampling**. With this method, individuals have an equal probability of being chosen and are selected from a larger sampling frame using

---

Box 2.1   A note on categorical and continuous data

Categorical data refer to counts in categories or classes. They are usually presented in tabular form such as:

	Exposed to known carcinogen	Not exposed to known carcinogen
Cancer present	7	5
Cancer not present	27	29

Each value in each *cell* of the table represents a count of people who have the characteristic defined by that cell's row and column. In the above, the count of 27, for example, represents 27 people who do not have cancer but have been exposed to a known carcinogen. Such data are often also termed *nominal* data.

Continuous data provide an exact position on a continuous scale and are not represented as counts in categories. Examples include a person's height (m) or weight (kg), the number of deaths from a certain cause per year in a region (deaths per year), toxic emissions from a factory chimney (tonnes per year) or the amount spent by a company on health and safety training (£ per year). A researcher has much more analytical scope with continuous data but may decide to convert it to nominal to aid in its description or summary.

THE DESIGN AND ANALYSIS OF EPIDEMIOLOGICAL STUDIES

EPIDEMIOLOGICAL INFORMATION

Data are the very life-blood of epidemiology. Epidemiologists can
that have been collected and published by others (**secondary d**
collect their own data by conducting surveys, for example (**pr**
data). There is a wide range of survey techniques and research
that can be used to collect data. The research designs are described
2 of the book. In this chapter we present a brief review of survey
but aim primarily to provide a review of sources of routine sec
health-related data. We also present an assessment of the value and
tions of routine sources and give some consideration to the second
of social surveys that collect health-related data.

At the end of the chapter you should:

- have an appreciation of the range of routine secondary data av
  for epidemiological research;
- understand the limitations and drawbacks of such data.

Collecting epidemiological data

The research designs which we go on to consider in the rest of Part
vide the basic frameworks for the collection of epidemiological data
mechanical and operational sense, however, the collection of epiden
gical data depends on survey methods. Here we use the term 'survey
broadly to contain not only questionnaires completed by an indivi
either in their right or by someone acting on their behalf, but also the
instruments which have been devised for the collection of routine inform
about health-related events such as the use of a hospital or the registra

---

Box 2.2   Survey coding

Q1: Is the respondent dead or alive?
Q2: Did the respondent smoke regularly (defined in detail) in 1984?

Coding stage

Respondent	Outcome (1 = dead)	Exposure (1 = smoker)
1	0	0
2	1	0
3	0	1
⋮	⋮	⋮
1224	1	1

Analysis stage
A. *Tally*: How many died? How many smoked? Counts of 0 or 1 in each column.
B. *Tabulation*: Code counts in cells.

	Died	Survived
Smoker	Code 1 for Outcome Code 1 for Exposure	Code 0 for Outcome Code 1 for Exposure
Non-smoker	Code 1 for Outcome Code 0 for Exposure	Code 0 for Outcome Code 0 for Exposure

C. *Full result of tabulation*

	Died	Survived	Total
Smoker	88	362	450
Non-smoker	92	682	774
Total	180	1044	1224

random numbers generated by computer or some random process such as coin-tossing. Where membership of some particular population subgroup or **stratum** is important for a study, for instance age grouping, people can be randomly sampled from a defined stratum in proportion to the size of the stratum. When the sampling process is not random there is a risk that systematic bias will occur (see Chapter 4). Clearly, too, the size of the **sample** matters; there needs to be a trade-off between having enough to discern patterns within the data, and wasting resources by collecting too many data. A range of websites provide ready access to software for sample size calculations.[1]

- **Coding**: the process of coding data refers to the assigning of a number to each response to each question. Qualitative statements (for example, a cause of death) need to be reduced to categories to which a code can be attached. Quantitative information can be entered as it stands (for example, raw age), summarized in bandings (for example, age bands) or summarized as category (for example, 1 = dead, 0 = survived). Box 2.1 explains the distinction between **continuous data** and categorical data. Box 2.2 summarizes the coding process for categorical data. It presents an extract of the individual survey responses from a major social survey. For each respondent there is an outcome (dead or not) and exposure indicator (smoker or not). The survey was completed by a member of a cohort of 1224 people or by a relative if the individual had died. The final cross-tabulation indicates that 88 of the cohort were smokers who had died.

Secondary routine data

Box 2.3 describes the key features of secondary data sources. When using data for secondary purposes it is particularly important to assess its quality and validity given that it is being used for a different purpose from that for which it was originally intended. There are four dimensions of quality that should be considered: accuracy, completeness, timeliness, and fitness of purpose. Three types of secondary data source are considered in this chapter: population, mortality and morbidity data.[2] In the concluding section of this chapter brief consideration is given to compendia sources and record linkage. In introducing each data source, consideration is given to the following:

- how the data are collected
- how the data are classified (where appropriate)
- quality and validity
- availability.

Population data

Population data are very important in enabling one to describe the size and key characteristics of a population and providing a *denominator* when calculating mortality and morbidity rates. The number of patients with a given condition, often referred to as the number of cases, provides important information for describing patterns of illness. Knowing the number of cases is an important starting point when considering the health of the

1 See, for example, http://www.psycholgie.uni-trier.de:8000/projects/gpower.html, or http://www.stat.ucla.edu/calculators/powercalc, or arguably the market-leader http://www.statsol.ie/nquery.html

2 Sources of official health-related data produced by the Government Statistical Service can be searched using StatBase® available over the World Wide Web at http://www.statistics.gov.uk/statbase/mainmenu.asp

---

Box 2.3 Features of secondary data

Secondary data are:

- routinely collected, collated and presented on a regular basis;
- collected for a particular (primary) purpose and subsequently made available for additional (secondary) purposes;
- typically used in descriptive studies.

---

population. However, it is difficult to make meaningful comparisons between different populations, geographical areas or time periods without knowledge of the underlying population being considered. Information is needed about whether study populations are similar in terms of their size and composition. Rates are used to adjust (control) for differences in the size of populations amongst the areas or subgroups being compared. In calculating rates, the population provides the denominator, and the number with or without a condition (for example, morbidity or mortality data) provides the *numerator* (see Box 2.4). Rates and standardization techniques are described in more detail in the next chapter.

Box 2.4 Rates

$$\text{Rate} = \frac{\text{Numerator}}{\text{Denominator}}$$

$$\text{Mortality rate} = \frac{\text{Number of people who have died}}{\text{Total population}}$$

$$\text{Morbidity rate} = \frac{\text{Number of people who have an illness}}{\text{Total population}}$$

The rate is often expressed as the number of cases per 1000 or 100,000 population; sometimes it is expressed as a percentage.

The population census

A national **census** typically involves a total enumeration of the population (head count). Since 1801 a *decennial* census has been undertaken – every ten years – in England and Wales (with the exception of 1941 owing to the Second World War). Every householder is legally required to complete a census questionnaire. The census not only provides appropriate denominator data for calculating rates but also includes key demographic details (age and sex) and information about socioeconomic characteristics such as occupation and socioeconomic class, and also information on household accommodation and amenities (Dale and Marsh 1993). Data are also collected on car ownership and are potentially useful given that

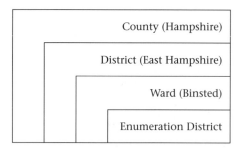

Figure 2.1   Hierarchical reference system used to identify census units.
Source: based on Martin 1991.

lack of personal transport can affect householders' ability to access certain
health care services (Joseph and Phillips 1984).

Census data are available for a number of geographical areas including
counties, health authorities, local authority districts and also small areas
known as wards and **enumeration districts** (EDs) (Cole 1993). The
relationship between some of these areas is shown in Figure 2.1. Census
data provide national coverage and near-complete enumeration of the
population (Dale and Marsh 1993). In summary, using census data it is
possible to:

● use it as a denominator with other health statistics and calculate
  disease-specific mortality/morbidity rates;
● describe the demography of an area;
● explore the nature of relationships between health and socioeconomic
  variables (housing tenure, amenities and occupational status).

For the first time ever, the 1991 census also included a question on
morbidity and this was asked directly of every person in each household
(Gould and Jones 1996). The exact wording of this question was: 'Does
the person have any long-term illness, health problem or handicap which
limits his/her activities or the work he/she can do?' (OPCS/RGO(S) 1991).
Using these data it is possible to calculate rates of general 'self-reported'
long-term limiting illness. Dale (1993a) notes that pre-census tests of the
limiting long-term illness data correlated well with other data on GP consultations and inpatient and outpatient visits to hospital and she argues
that this measure of self-reported morbidity provides the only nationally
consistent indicator of health service needs.

A number of indices have been developed which seek to combine census variables into a single measure of deprivation (Townsend *et al.* 1988;
Jarman 1983; Senior 1991). Numerous studies have shown associations
between these deprivation measures and health status.

In the UK census, validation exercises are undertaken by the ONS
(Office for National Statistics formerly OPCS, Office of Population Censuses and Surveys) to evaluate both the coverage and the quality of census
responses (Wiggins 1993). It was estimated that there were 1 million
missing people not enumerated in the 1991 census accounted for mainly
by a 1 per cent shortfall in the number of men aged 19–31 (Marsh 1993a:

Table 2.1 Principal census data outputs

Outputs	England and Wales	Scotland	Northern Ireland
Printed volumes (available in many libraries)			
National monitors	✔	✔	
National summary reports	✔	✔	✔
County monitors	✔	✔	
County reports	✔	✔	
Computer-readable data			
County monitors	✔	✔	
County reports	✔	✔	
Local base statistics	✔	✔	
Small area statistics	✔	✔	✔
ED/postcode directory	✔	✔	✔
SARs (Sample of Anonymized Records)	✔	✔	✔
Longitudinal survey	✔		

Source: Dale and Marsh 1993.

157; Charlton and Murphy 1997). It has been suggested that this shortfall was linked to avoidance of community charge payments (Charlton and Murphy 1997: 8). There are also some other inaccuracies with census data and these are due to transcription and coding errors (Wiggins 1993). Overall, the accuracy and completeness of national censuses is felt to be very good. The main limitation with data is that they quickly become out of date and disaggregate output is not made available until two years after the census (although faster distribution is promised for the 2001 census). Despite these concerns, census data are central to developing an understanding of the demography of an area and are used extensively by health authorities to develop profiles of their localities (Portsmouth and South East Hampshire Health Authority 1990, 1996).

Census data are made available in a number of different formats (Table 2.1). A series of national and county reports and monitors are published that provide detailed tables and key statistics (Denham 1993). These reports do not contain data disaggregated for areas smaller than local authority districts. Topic-based reports (for example, limiting long-term illness, housing and availability of cars) are also produced but generally do not contain statistics that are disaggregated geographically. Machine-readable data are available for a variety of small areas: wards and enumeration districts (EDs). These data outputs are known as the local base statistics (LBS) and the small area statistics (SAS) (Cole 1993). Data are also made available electronically for other geographical units including standard regions, counties, local authority districts, health authorities, old regional health authorities (RHAs) and postcode areas.

The LBS/SAS contain a very large number of tables (Table 2.2), although these only contain cross-tabulations of a small number of variables. For example, it is not possible to cross-tabulate the illness question with more than three other demographic and socioeconomic variables (Gould and

Table 2.2 Contents of census LBS

Themes	LBS tables
Demographic and economic characteristics	1–18
Housing	19–27
Households and household composition	28–53
Household spaces and dwellings	54–66
Tables for Scotland and Wales	67–70
10% topics on employment and occupation (difficult to code)	71–99

Source: OPCS User Guide 38; Dale and Marsh 1993: Appendix 8.1.

Jones 1996). The LBS/SAS was purchased centrally for health service use and health authorities can use it freely for any activity, as long as this is at least half NHS funded (Denham 1993). The data were also purchased for the academic sector, and students and university researchers can use them freely for academic purposes. A CD-ROM produced under licence by Chadwyck Healey Ltd provides easy access to the census LBS/SAS and can be found in some libraries. Census data are most frequently extracted and manipulated using the SASPAC software package designed for this purpose (Davies 1995). Academic users can access the data over the internet using the MIMAS (Manchester Information and Associated Services) system.[3] CASWEB provides a very easy to use web-based interface for extracting census data[4] (Martin *et al*. 1998). Strict licensing agreements govern all use of census data and exist to protect individual privacy and Crown copyright.

A number of other statistical abstracts and census-related products are also available as summarized in Table 2.1 (Dale and Marsh 1993). The Sample of Anonymised Records (SARs) contains non-identifiable census responses for samples of individuals and households and provides a valuable source of 'microdata' (Marsh 1993b; Gould and Jones 1996). Digital boundary data for wards, EDs and other geographical areas can be used to display census data in map form. An ED/postcode directory is also available which allows the user to determine for a particular address which ED it is most likely to be located within. This also facilitates the production of 'user defined' areas for data analysis (Martin 1991).

The Longitudinal Survey

The Longitudinal Survey (LS) has followed a 1 per cent sample of the population who share one of four dates of birth since the 1971 census (Dale 1993b; Hattersley and Creeser 1995). New births and immigrants who share these birth dates are also added to the LS database. A number of data records held by the ONS for each LS member are linked together. These include census records (for 1971, 1981 and 1991); 'vital events' (including live births, still births, deaths, infant deaths, deaths of spouses); cancer registrations; entry into psychiatric hospital (until 1984); and emigration and re-entry (SSRU 1990). Detailed demographic and socioeconomic

3 Further information can be found at http://www.mimas.ac.uk/
4 This can be accessed at http://census.ac.uk/casweb/

cross-tabulations and multivariate analyses can be requested through the LS User Support Programme.[5] A number of longitudinal and cross-sectional analyses are possible, including analysis of:

- relationships between morbidity, chronic illness and mortality;
- household patterns in health;
- geographical variations in health;
- patterns and trends through time.

Population estimates and projections

The national census only provides a 'snapshot' of the population every ten years and for many purposes it is important to have regularly updated population estimates. The term **population estimate** is used to describe an estimate of the population based between censuses and makes use of what is known about births, deaths (see next section) and migration patterns – all of which are recorded on the NHS Central Register (Fox 1990). A simplified outline of one common method used to produce population estimates is shown in Box 2.5. Fuller detail can be found in Marsh (1993a: table 6.9).

Box 2.5   Population estimates

These are made by:

- taking baseline population data from the census
- deducting the number of deaths known to have occurred during the year(s) under consideration
- adding the number of births
- adding the number of immigrants
- making adjustments for the age distribution.

Population projections are produced by extrapolating population data using known patterns of births, deaths and migration to predicted future figures. In other words the key difference between population estimates and projections is that the former are based on known levels of births, deaths and migration, whilst the latter are made on the basis of predicted future levels. Both are useful in helping to plan services by giving some idea of current and future population size and composition.

The ONS produces national and subnational (including health authority) population estimates and projections regularly. These are available in paper format and are summarized in Table 2.3 (see also OPCS 1992a, b). Many local authorities in England and Wales produce ward-based population estimates (Rees 1994; Simpson *et al.* 1997; Simpson 1998). The accuracy of the estimates and projections will depend upon the methodology used and also the quality of the data used. The registration of births and deaths is a legal requirement and ensures high quality data. Information on the numbers

---

5 Based at the Centre for Longitudinal Studies, Institute of Education, University of London. Further information is available at http://www.cls.ioe.ac.uk/Ls/lshomepage.html.

of immigrants and emigrants are likely to be less reliable as they are dependent upon individuals registering with a GP. Population projections for small areas are likely to be inaccurate as it is difficult to make estimates for areas that are changing rapidly, and also those that have large numbers of students and members of the armed forces (Simpson *et al.* 1997).

Vital statistics

The term **vital events** relates to births, deaths and marriages, and the Births, Marriages and Deaths Act 1839 requires their notification to a local registrar within six weeks of occurrence. The ONS collates and publishes this information as vital statistics (Table 2.3). We first consider birth statistics and then go on to consider mortality statistics.

Table 2.3 Routine statistical publications produced by the ONS

Series	Topic
Population data	
PP1	*Mid-year Population Estimates*
PP2	*National Population Projections*
PP3	*Sub-national Population Projections*
Vital statistics	
VS1	*Vital Statistics Summary (Population, Births, Deaths, Fertility and Mortality Rates)*
VS2	*Birth Statistics*
VS3	*Mortality Statistics (Deaths by Cause, Age and Sex)*
VS4	*Vital Statistics for Wards (Births and Deaths)*
VS4D	*Deaths from Selected Causes by Wards*
VS5	*Infant Mortality*
FM1	*Birth Statistics*
Death data	
DH1	*Mortality Statistics: General*
DH2	*Mortality Statistics: Cause*
DH3	*Mortality Statistics: Childhood, Infant and Perinatal*
DH4	*Mortality Statistics: Injury and Poisoning*
DH5	*Mortality Statistics: Area*
DH6	*Mortality Statistics: Childhood*
DS	*Decennial Supplements*
Morbidity statistics	
MB1	*Cancer Statistics: Registrations*
MB2	*Communicable Disease Statistics*
MB3	*Congenital Anomaly Statistics*
MB4	*Hospital In-patient Enquiry*
MB5	*Morbidity Statistics from General Practice*
MB6	*Key Health Statistics from General Practice*
Miscellaneous statistics	
AB	*Abortion Statistics*

All these publications are published by The Stationery Office (further details at //http://www.the-stationery-office.co.uk and //http:/www.ukstate.com)

Births

All births in the UK must be registered at the local Registry of Births, Deaths and Marriages by either the parent(s) or a representative of the parent(s). Some of the information collected at registration is publicly available: child's name, sex, date of birth; mother's name, place of birth and usual place of residence; father's name (if known), father's place of birth and occupation. Additional, confidential data are collected for statistical purposes: parents' dates of birth, and in the case of births within marriage, date of marriage and the number of children born to the mother in previous marriages. Stillbirths are registered in the same way as live births but an additional cause of death certificate is completed by the attending registered medical practitioner or the midwife involved in the pregnancy. Given that registration is mandatory, birth statistics have near complete coverage. There is some delay in publishing the statistics, although data for a particular calendar year are generally made available one year later. Vital statistics are made available by ONS to health and local authority organizations in paper form (Table 2.3) and more recently also in computer disc format.

Mortality information

Epidemiologists would like to be able to determine levels of ill health (morbidity) amongst a population to identify those who need to be treated in an effort to improve the nation's health and reduce premature deaths. Often, however, secondary data relating to morbidity are not available, so mortality data, which are more readily available, are used as a proxy for determining levels of disease. Death is a 'vital event' and must be registered by a 'qualified informant' – typically a relative of the deceased who can provide information about date and place of death, date and place of birth, occupation, usual address and occupation. Figure 2.2 summarizes the steps involved in registering a death in England and Wales.

A dead body cannot be legally buried or cremated in the UK without a death certificate. The medical practitioner who last attended the deceased (during their final illness) is required to identify the *underlying* cause of death. If a medical practitioner was not present, a coroner is required to conduct an inquest to establish the events leading up to death. The medical

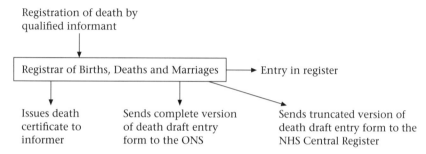

Figure 2.2 Summary of death registration procedures in England and Wales. *Source*: SSRU 1990.

Table 2.4 Basic categories in ICD-10

Chapter	Disease categories	Range of codes	Example
I	Certain infectious and parasitic diseases	A00-B99	Malaria
II	Neoplasms	C00-D48	Malignant neoplasm of larynx
III	Disease of the blood and blood forming organs and certain disorders involving the immune mechanism	D50-D89	Anaemia
IV	Endocrine, nutritional and metabolic diseases	E00-E90	Diabetes Mellitus
V	Mental and behavioural disorders	F00-F99	Paranoid schizophrenia
VI	Diseases of the nervous system	G00-G99	Epilepsy
VII	Diseases of the eye and adnexa	H00-H59	
VIII	Diseases of the ear and mastoid process	H60-H95	
IX	Diseases of the circulatory system	I00-I99	Hypertension
X	Diseases of the respiratory system	J00-J99	Acute bronchitis
XI	Diseases of the digestive system	K00-K93	Appendicitis
XII	Disease of the skin and subcutaneous tissue	L00-L99	Dermatitis
XIII	Diseases of the musculo-skeletal system and connective tissue	M00-M99	Rheumatoid arthritis
XIV	Disease of the genito-urinary system	N00-N99	Acute renal failure
XV	Pregnancy, childbirth and the puerperium	O00-O99	Postpartum haemorrhage
XVI	Certain conditions originating in the perinatal period	P00-P95	Slow foetal growth
XVII	Congenital malformations, deformations, and chromosomal abnormalities	Q00-Q99	Spina bifida
XVIII	Symptoms, signs and abnormal clinical and laboratory findings, not elsewhere classified	R00-R99	Sudden death, cause unknown
XIX	Injury, poisoning and certain other consequences of external causes	S00-T98	Poisoning by psychotropic drugs
XX	External causes of morbidity and mortality	V01-Y98	Intentional self-harm by hanging
XXI	Factors influencing health status and contact with health services	Z00-Z98	Threat of job loss

Source: WHO (1992).

certificate used in England and Wales is similar to that recommended by the World Health Organization (WHO) and provides for the separate identification of conditions which lead directly to death and other significant conditions present which may have contributed to death. There is a separate neonatal death certificate form for deaths occurring during the first 28 days of life and the attending medical practitioner is required to distinguish between foetal and maternal contributions to the cause of death.

The registrar sends the information to the ONS where it is coded and entered onto computer. The deceased's postcode is added and the cause of death is coded using the *International Classification of Disease* (ICD). The tenth revision of this classification (ICD-10) is in the process of being introduced in the UK. It makes use of an alphanumeric coding system rather than the purely numerical system used in ICD-9 and provides a larger number of categories for classification. The summary codes for ICD-10 are shown in Table 2.4.

The VS3 series gives detail of death by cause, age and sex for local authority areas; whilst VS4 series provides ward-level data. Additionally, the ONS publishes the DH series of annual national reports on mortality for England and Wales. For example, the ONS publication *Mortality Statistics by Cause* (DH2) provides statistics on the numbers of deaths and standardized mortality rates (see Chapter 3) for selected causes of death. The ONS also publishes a series of decennial supplements (the DS series) focused on mortality and geography (Britton 1990; OPCS n.d., 1990); occupational health (Drever 1995); children's health (Botting 1995); and the health of adults (Charlton and Murphy 1997); and have produced life tables that show the numbers of people surviving to a particular age and the life expectancy for people of a particular age (ONS 1997a). The DS series makes use of mortality statistics aggregated for a number of years and thus eliminates the problems of chance fluctuations in disease incidence associated with rare conditions (Chilvers 1978; Leck 1989). The series also relates mortality data to the population enumerated at the last census, thereby providing a more reliable denominator for the calculation of mortality rates than those used for data published on an annual basis (Alderson 1987).

Data coverage regarding mortality is generally accepted as complete, but errors can occur in one or more of the many processes which lead to the publishing of mortality statistics. There are particular problems associated with the accuracy of death registration and certification (Prior 1985). In some cases it may be difficult for the medical practitioner to identify the underlying cause(s) of death; whilst the distinction between immediate cause of death, other significant conditions and underlying cause is not always easily made. If the practitioner uses non-standard terminology for the cause of death on the certificate this will result in problems in assigning codes. In general, death certificates are less precise for the elderly as there are likely to be a range underlying factors and causes that have contributed to eventual death.

Morbidity

Morbidity data provide information on patterns and variation in (ill)health, and are more useful than mortality data when wanting to describe and analyse current trends in illness. After all, the data deal with people who are still alive. There are, however, great difficulties inherent in using morbidity data. First, there is a general lack of availability (although the situation has improved throughout the 1990s). Secondly, the recording of morbidity data is generally dependent on patients presenting themselves to a health service professional and recognizing that they are ill. It will be biased by tolerance to pain and discomfort, willingness to seek assistance, and also cultural factors and beliefs. In some instances, patients may seek assistance from alternative complementary therapists or from private health care providers. Neither of these contributes to the secondary data sources routinely collected by the government statistical service. Thirdly, and as with mortality, problems occur with respect to the diagnosis and subsequent classification of illness. The quality and coverage of morbidity data are thus highly variable. Consideration is given here to following sources of morbidity data:

- Morbidity Statistics from General Practice
- **notification** of infectious diseases
- cancer registrations
- notification of sexually transmitted diseases
- **hospital activity data**
- congenital malformations.

Morbidity Statistics from General Practice (MSGP)

The Royal College of General Practitioners (RCGP) carries out a national study of morbidity and the results are published by the ONS. The study is based on a sample of volunteer practices and information is collected on consultations and disease. The results are biased, as 'study' practices are self-selecting and tend to be 'different' from other practices throughout England and Wales. The practices tend to have a larger than average patient list, younger partners, and GPs interested in research (OPCS 1995). The General Practice Research Database (GPRD) provides a partial complement to the data from the MSGP. A general practice computer software company (VAMP) set up the GPRD although it is now managed by the ONS on behalf of the Department of Health (ONS 1996). GPRD, like MSGP, is reliant on volunteer practices but does cover 6 per cent of the population in England and Wales and provides prevalence rates for selected conditions. The RCGP also produces a Weekly Return Service which records new episodes of illness seen in the GP practices that took part in the 1991/92 MSGP.

Notification of infectious diseases

Medical personnel (in general practice and hospitals) are required to notify their local 'proper officer' of any cases of infectious disease that they identify. The ONS and the Communicable Disease Surveillance Centre (CDSC) (part of the Public Health Laboratory Service) are subsequently informed of all incidents of notifiable diseases. In some cases a blood or faeces sample is taken from the patient and sent away for laboratory analysis to confirm diagnosis. Diseases requiring notification include relatively mild childhood infections such as rubella (German measles), food poisoning, dysentery, and rarer tropical diseases like Lassa fever. Despite the notification of some infectious diseases attracting a target payment for medical practitioners, notifications are far from complete. The formal notification process can be validated against data from the Public Health Laboratory Service (see Chapter 10). The ONS produces quarterly and annual monitors on communicable diseases.

Cancer registrations

Since 1962, all hospitals in England and Wales have joined a voluntary national registration scheme. The scheme is dependent on clinics and hospitals cooperating with Regional Cancer Registries in the collection of data. All registered cancer patients are flagged and tracked on the NHS Central Register (Fox 1990) until they die and this allows survival statistics (time to death) to be calculated. There is some evidence to suggest that the registration of cancer is fairly complete although the accuracy of cancer statistics is of some concern. Whilst diagnosis is typically accurate, there are errors associated with the date of registration, histology and occupation (if collected). The ONS produces an annual monitor which reports on statistics relating to cancer registrations. Regular reports are also produced by Regional Cancer Registries and some international comparisons of cancer statistics are also available (Mould 1983).

Notification of sexually transmitted diseases

Regular statistical returns about new cases of sexually transmitted disease (STD) are sent by genito-urinary medicine (GUM) clinics to the Department of Health so that national trends can be identified. These returns do not include notifications of HIV and AIDS as these are reported to the director of CDSC using a separate and confidential reporting system.

Hospital activity

Data are routinely collected within hospital settings relating to clinical activity. These data became important in supporting the contracting process when the providers and purchasers of health care in the NHS were separated in the early 1990s (Wrigley 1991; More and Martin 1998). In the NHS, there is a diverse range of clinical information to support specific specialities but the recording and coverage of routine activity data are currently limited by nationally defined minimum basic datasets. It should be noted when utilizing these data that there is currently no reliable routinely available public source detailing activity undertaken within private hospitals apart from that activity which is paid for by the NHS. To date, coverage of inpatient hospital activity is also far more complete than that for day cases or outpatient activity.

Routinely collected inpatient information includes a patient's basic demographic and medical details, details of the hospital treatment process (for example, type of admission, duration of stay), and diagnostic information. Diagnoses are now classified according to ICD-10 and operative procedures use the OPCS4 classification. The move to the former creates problems in analysing time trends, whilst the latter is outdated and fails to identify many modern interventions. There are ongoing debates about other systems for classifying hospital activity. The accuracy and completeness of diagnostic and operative coding are improving but still need to be considered when using hospital activity data.

Since the late 1980s the key unit of measurement has been **finished consultant episodes** (FCEs) which reflect the work undertaken by consultants. FCEs measure hospital activity and not disease episodes. Caution must thus be taken when using these statistics as a proxy for morbidity. The grouping of FCEs to produce more homogeneous clinical and statistical categories provides a means of reducing the large number of categories to be considered. Such groupings are provided by the HRGs (**Healthcare Resource Groups**) produced by the National Casemix Office. Summary tables of (hospital) activity data are published in paper and electronic form (Government Statistical Service 1995, 1996a, b, c). Individual records can be obtained in electronic format from a number of sources including local NHS Trust hospital information systems and health authority district information systems.

Congenital malformations

Following the thalidomide scandal in 1960 a national scheme was initiated in 1964 to enable notifications of congenital malformation. The doctor or midwife notifying the birth is asked to include particulars of any congenital malformation together with information about live/still birth, place of birth, length of gestation, birth weight, multiple birth, mother's date of birth. Anecdotal evidence suggests that the data are not complete and levels of reporting vary depending upon the type of malformation.

Social surveys

The morbidity data sources described in the previous section are all derived from official routine sources, and collected for administrative and clinical purposes. They result from patients presenting themselves to a health professional. Minor illnesses and other conditions not associated with a consultation are unlikely to be included in these sources and such information can usually only be obtained by employing the survey methods described briefly at the start of this chapter. The question on self-reported morbidity contained in the 1991 census provides a partial exception to this position.

The General Household Survey (GHS), undertaken by the ONS, provides a rich socioeconomic data source with the ability to cross-tabulate health data against a range of other variables. The exact content of the GHS varies from year to year, though each annual report gives details of the topics covered and the questionnaire used (ONS 1998). Examples of health-related topics considered over the past 30 years include: drinking and smoking behaviour, fertility, chronic and acute sickness, general health, hospital outpatient attendees, accidents, dental health, sight and hearing and use of walking aids.

More recently, the Department of Health has commissioned an annual Health Survey for England to provide more regular information about aspects of people's health and to monitor some of the *Health of the Nation* targets (Prescott-Clarke and Primatesta 1996). The British Household Panel Survey (BHPS), established in 1991, has a longitudinal design where the original interviewees are followed up through time and re-interviewed during successive 'waves' of the survey (Buck *et al.* 1994; Rose *et al.* 1994). The BHPS has included questions on smoking, health, income and wealth, socioeconomic factors, housing and household composition.

The Health and Lifestyle Survey (HALS) is a comprehensive survey of the physical and mental health, and health-related behaviour of a sample of 9003 individuals initially interviewed in 1984/85 (Cox *et al.* 1987). Although the original study was designed as a cross-sectional survey, attempts were made to re-interview during 1991/92. HALS contains data on smoking, alcohol, eating and exercise, blood pressure and mental health as well as the usual demographic and socioeconomic confounders. The data have been found to be highly representative of the national population (Blaxter 1990). The original respondents have also been subsequently 'flagged' on the NHS Central Register to obtain information on both the date and cause of death and this is known as the HALS Death Data (Cox 1995).

All these national surveys have associated published reports that provide commentaries and aggregated results. Academic researchers can obtain anonymized individual-based data through the national Data Archive based at the University of Essex. The relative design merits of each of these surveys need to be considered to ensure appropriate interpretation and analysis (Twigg 1999). In addition to these surveys there are number of other longitudinal birth cohort studies that have studied and followed newly born babies through childhood and adulthood. They provide information on child development, health-related behaviour, education, socioeconomic status, and hopes and aspirations (Ekinsmyth 1996).

Conclusion

In addition to the sources described above, it is not uncommon for local initiatives to lead to the establishment of disease registers and the collation of datasets which focus on a particular condition. Disease registers are also held by local health organizations and voluntary organizations (for example the Stroke Association). Local authorities sometimes maintain databases which contain details about disabled clients. These sources are often ad hoc in nature and access may be difficult and dependent on having local contacts. Moreover, use will require guarantees from users that the confidentiality of individuals will be maintained and approval from a Local Research Ethics Committee if the data originated within the NHS.

There are also a number of compendia sources containing health information which provide summaries of selected data from many of the sources described above. The *Public Health Common Data Set* (PHCDS) is produced annually by the National Institute of Epidemiology at the University of Surrey on behalf of the Department of Health. It provides a wide range of health indicators, demography, fertility, morbidity and mortality, and allows comparisons to be made between health authorities. In recent years the dataset has been expanded to include *Health of the Nation Monitoring Indicators* and *Public Health Outcome Indicators* (DoH/NIE 1996).

Finally, it is worth noting that many researchers and agencies have attempted to link different health-related datasets together using record linkage techniques (Baldwin *et al.* 1987). Jones *et al.* (1991) link records contained in a call–recall and vaccination appointment system and a child health surveillance information system to undertake a multilevel statistical analysis of child immunization uptake. Other researchers have flagged individuals on the NHS Central Register to track individuals and undertake survival analysis (Fox 1990). A pilot study undertaken in Oxford in 1967 which linked birth, hospital discharge and death data provides another early and notable example (Acheson 1967).

This chapter has reviewed a number of routine secondary data sources and health surveys used by epidemiologists. Many of these data sources are used in the day-to-day work of district epidemiologists (Chapter 10). In using secondary data sources, detailed consideration should be given to data quality and validity. In particular, issues of bias and representativeness need to be borne in mind.

Summary

- Epidemiologists use data that have been collected and published by others (secondary data) or collect their own data by conducting surveys. Conducting a good survey is difficult. Secondary data are readily available but may not address your specific research needs. It is important to understand the limitations and drawbacks of epidemiological data and their sources.

- Census data provide national coverage and near-complete enumeration of the population. They are widely used in epidemiology as a denominator in the calculation of disease-specific mortality/morbidity rates.

- Vital statistics cover matters to do with birth and death. These topics are the subject of statutory registration requirements so the data are generally accurate.

- Morbidity data provide information on patterns and variation in (ill)health, and are more useful than mortality data when wanting to describe and analyse current trends in illness. The quality and coverage of morbidity data are highly variable.

- Data from large-scale social surveys provide a rich socioeconomic data source with the ability to cross-tabulate health data against a range of other variables. Academic researchers can obtain anonymized individual-based data through the national Data Archive based at the University of Essex.

Further reading

Dale, A. and Marsh, C. (eds) (1993) *The 1991 Census User's Guide*. London: HMSO.

Dorling, D. and Simpson, S. (eds) (1999) *Statistics in Society*. London: Arnold (Part V and especially chapter 26).

Radical Statistics Health Group (1999) *Official Health Statistics: An Unofficial Guide*. London: Arnold.

Activities

1 One of the most notoriously difficult areas in which to conduct epidemiological survey work is that of health-related behaviour. Imagine you have been asked to conduct a survey on patterns of 'unhealthy eating' in relation to heart disease. You are limited to eight questions. What questions would you include and how would you word them? Remember that you will need to identify subgroups in the population as well as ask about unhealthy eating. When you have devised your questionnaire, try it out on a colleague and seek critical feedback.

2 Your local NHS library or university library should be able to point you in the direction of collections of routine statistics. Try to find out the following:

(a) Which local government wards in your home town or nearest town have the highest and lowest percentages of people with limiting long-term illness?

(b) Which local government wards in your home town or nearest town have the highest and lowest percentages of people who are out of work?

(c) How many babies were born in your local district/unitary authority last year?

(d) What are the four most common causes of death in the UK? How does this vary between age groups?

You will need to work out which source of data is most appropriate for each of these questions.

3 Try to access a copy of ICD-10. Choose a disease of interest to you and try to work out which ICD codes might be involved.

PATTERNS OF DISEASE

This chapter introduces the ways in which epidemiological studies are put together. It considers the most basic of all epidemiological study designs, and it will consider how patterns in the incidence and prevalence of disease can be described. The chapter begins by extending our discussion of the key features of descriptive epidemiology. It then looks at the concepts central to what are known as **cross-sectional (or prevalence) studies**. A case study of ischaemic heart disease is presented in order to exemplify these concepts.

At the end of this chapter you should:

● understand the key elements of descriptive epidemiology;
● understand the strengths and weaknesses of prevalence (cross-sectional) approaches to looking at disease;
● appreciate the analytical issues involved in cross-sectional studies;
● be aware of the value of even these simple approaches to understanding disease and planning health care services.

Descriptive epidemiology

As noted in Chapter 1, descriptive epidemiology is concerned with identifying patterns in diseases. The intention of a descriptive study is to provide an overview of a particular problem. Descriptive studies are concerned with addressing questions such as:

- How big a problem is a particular disease or condition?
- Is the incidence or prevalence of the condition increasing over time?
- How does incidence or prevalence vary from one area to another?
- Which people are most or least affected by the condition?

An important characteristic of descriptive epidemiological studies is that they are often based on *secondary* data. These are data that are not collected by the end-user. Chapter 2 outlined key sources of health data that are collected routinely and discussed the validity of those sources. The quality of descriptive epidemiological studies is highly dependent on the data upon which they are based and, when these are secondary data, the epidemiologist can have little or no influence on the quality of the input data. On the other hand, a study based on routine data can be undertaken rapidly and relatively cheaply compared with studies that require collection of primary data.

The starting point of a descriptive study should be a clear definition of the condition to be described (Farmer *et al.* 1996). This will usually include an explicit statement of subconditions which are to be included in the study, any exclusions, and details of the codes used to classify the condition. Information from existing studies of the size of the problem being investigated will also typically be included. This gives justification to undertaking an inquiry. Mortality and morbidity rates are usually used to establish the size of the problem.

The core of a descriptive study is the analysis of mortality or morbidity data to identify variations on three axes: time, place and person. Two distinct types of variation in terms of *time* might be identified: long-term trends in the incidence or prevalence of a disease over time, and cyclical changes such as might result from seasonal variation in incidence or prevalence. *Place* variation can be identified at a number of different levels: between countries, between regions within countries and within specific institutions such as places of work or schools. *Person* characteristics that might be of interest are of two types. Age, sex and ethnic group are examples of intrinsic factors which might affect how likely somebody is to acquire a particular disease. Intrinsic factors are sometimes considered to be fixed as they refer to factors that cannot be prevented. The other group of personal characteristics of interest is those which increase an individual's risk of acquiring the condition under investigation. These are often referred to as lifestyle factors and include type of occupation, family and cultural factors. Lifestyle factors are also known as variable risk factors as they refer to potentially preventable factors.

Cross-sectional studies

Cross-sectional studies, also known as prevalence studies, are a particular type of descriptive study which are often used to identify variations in terms of person characteristics. A cross-sectional study involves selecting a sample of subjects and then determining the distribution of exposure and disease within that sample. Some studies may be highly descriptive, aiming to provide information only on the prevalence of a disease or an exposure in a population, hence the use of the term 'prevalence'. Cross-sectional studies can, however, be used analytically if associations are sought between exposure and health outcome. The key distinguishing feature is a single period of observation, the cross-section, in which both exposure and disease histories are collected simultaneously. This data collection can include a retrospective assessment of a history of disease or exposures.

Health care providers can use cross-sectional studies to assess the impact of a disease in a community, and to plan the distribution of medical resources. They can be used to calculate disease frequency for the population under study or for different subgroups within that population. Cross-sectional studies are thus an appropriate method for answering questions such as:

- Is migraine common in this community?
- What is the prevalence of dementia in elderly people?

In short, they are extremely useful for determining the 'burden of disease', that is, describing the magnitude and distribution of a health problem. They can also play a useful role in generating hypotheses about possible disease causation.

Farmer *et al.* (1996) provide an example of a cross-sectional study. These researchers sent postal questionnaires to a sample of households in England, Scotland and Wales. The 10,000 respondents, aged between 35 and 69 years, provided information on age, current smoking habits, place of residence and respiratory symptoms. The answers to the place of residence were used to estimate exposure to air pollution (high or low), while on the basis of the respiratory questions, the presence or absence of chronic bronchitis was determined. The prevalence of the disease increased with age and was generally lowest for non-smokers. The study can be criticized for not considering previous smoking habits and it is likely that current place of residence would give a fairly poor measure of a lifetime's exposure to pollution, especially pollution at work.

An important variant of the basic cross-sectional study is the **repeated cross-sectional study**. In this sort of study cross-sections of the population are asked the same questions on different occasions but no attempt is made to sample the same people in each repetition. We can gain some idea of how an issue of interest changes over time using the repeated cross-sectional approach. With this type of study it is, however, only possible to look at aggregate or net change because it is not the same individual who is repeatedly measured. Thus, while a repeated cross-sectional survey may show a slow overall decline in cigarette smoking, a true **panel study** (where the same individuals are asked the same question on each measurement occasion) may show a much more dynamic situation in which individuals are repeatedly quitting and starting smoking.

The Health Survey for England (HSE) is an example of a repeated cross-sectional study. The survey is commissioned by the Department of Health, was first undertaken in 1991, and since 1994 has been carried out by the

Joint Health Surveys Unit of Social and Community Planning Research (SCPR) and the Department of Epidemiology and Community Health, University College London. A sampling framework based on the national Postcode Address File is used to establish a representative sample of households which takes into account different kinds of area and household. Adults aged 16 and over in the selected households are interviewed and the interviewee is subsequently visited by a nurse who undertakes selected physiological measurements and takes a blood sample for further testing. The interviews are carried out throughout the year to reduce the effects of seasonal variations. Some 16,000 respondents are interviewed each year. The survey seeks to establish the prevalence of major conditions. Socioeconomic variables and lifestyle factors are also collected to enable examination of prevalence to be correlated with risk factors.

In summary, cross-sectional studies are useful when a 'snapshot' of disease prevalence is required. Participation can be high because little is demanded of the subjects. They are also relatively straightforward to do. They are, however, not the ideal design for studying diseases that are rare in the population: even a large survey may yield but few cases of rare diseases or diseases with short duration. Further limitations stem mainly from their lack of power for studies of disease **aetiology**. In aetiological prevalence studies it is often difficult to distinguish factors associated with risk of disease from factors associated with survival. Moreover, the simultaneous collection of exposure and disease histories can make for difficulties in working out which came first.

Data analysis in cross-sectional studies

Some of the data collected from cross-sectional studies will be continuous data (see Chapter 2). Continuous data analysis techniques are often used at the start of epidemiological studies to describe the basic characteristics of the study population such as its age or income profile. They are also important for *comparing* the characteristics of different study groups. For example, if a researcher was interested in comparing the effects of long working hours on overall health status, a comparison might be made between companies that schedule compulsory long breaks in the working period and those that had not introduced such a policy. The first task would be to use techniques of continuous data description to investigate the age profiles of each type of company.

There are many tools for continuous data description and analysis and many well written texts covering the subject area. The reader is advised to examine some of those available. Erickson and Nosanchuk (1992) and Marsh (1988), for example, provide very readable chapters on the exploration and description of continuous data.

One of the most common ways of summarizing continuous data is with the aid of a graphical tool called a *histogram*. The data are translated into frequency counts for ordered categories. Figure 3.1, for example, provides a histogram of respondent's age from the 1994 Health Survey for England. The horizontal axis (the *x*-axis) represents the age categories listed in

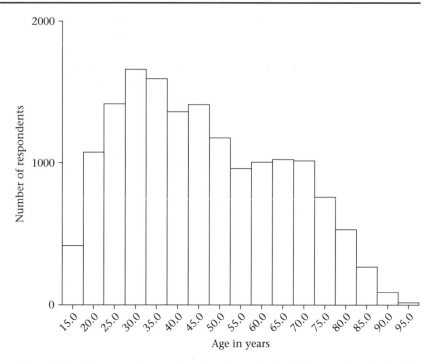

Figure 3.1   Histogram of respondents' age from the Health Survey of England 1994.

ascending order, and the *y*-axis represents the frequency count. Histograms are important for describing the *frequency distribution* or *frequency curve* of a variable and the overall shape of the graph will indicate where the typical or average value lies and how clustered the rest of the values are around this central value. These characteristics of a frequency curve are known as the *level* and *spread* respectively. Glancing at a spreadsheet of raw continuous data cannot easily assess such measures. A histogram, however, immediately provides information on the overall shape of the distribution. The graph in Figure 3.1, for example, indicates that the age distribution has a peak to the left-hand side of the graph for respondents aged between 25 and 45 years. Similar graphs could be constructed for males and females separately – or for any other social grouping – thus allowing comparisons of the distributions to be made.

A number of 'classic' frequency curve shapes are illustrated in Figure 3.2. The **normal (or Gaussian) curve** will be referred to later in this chapter. It is symmetrical about a single peak. More commonly, however, a variable may be negatively or positively skewed with a tail extending to the left- or right-hand side of the graph. As an example, weekly alcohol consumption, as recorded in the Health Survey of England, shows a highly positively skewed distribution. There are many people in England who do not consume alcohol at all and very many who drink only one or two units a week. The graph then tails off to extreme values to the right, where there is a small percentage of people consuming high quantities of alcohol on a weekly basis.

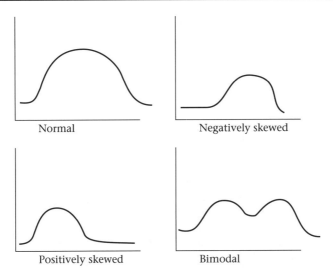

Figure 3.2 Classic frequency shapes.

Numerical measures can also be calculated to summarize the level and spread of a frequency distribution. As described above, the level refers to the 'centre' or typical value of a distribution whereas the spread indicates how clustered the rest of the values are around this typical value. There are several measures of both level and spread. The most commonly used are the **mean**, which is a measure of level and involves adding up all the values and dividing by the number of values, and the **standard deviation**, a measure that describes the average spread of all the values around the mean.

The arithmetic mean or average can be an inappropriate measure for certain types of frequency distribution. If the distribution is skewed, then the arithmetic average will be disproportionately affected by these extreme values and will no longer represent the typical values of the dataset.

Measures of spread are used to indicate whether other values are similar to the typical measure. A fairly compact distribution will have a correspondingly small spread measure. A wide range in the values will generate a big spread measure. Unusual values in a dataset can also heavily influence the standard deviation.

Prevalence and incidence

The notions of prevalence and incidence were introduced in Chapter 1. These measures are often used in descriptive designs where the emphasis is on investigating patterns of disease in relation to other variables such as time, place, and socioeconomic background. *Prevalence cases* are the number of existing cases of a disease or health condition in a specific population at some designated time. Thus there may be 503 asthmatics in the City of Portsmouth on 1 May 1999; two important types of prevalence proportion are recognized (Box 3.1A). **Point prevalence** is the proportion of a population known to have the disease at a particular time and **period**

Box 3.1   Prevalence and incidence measures

A. *Point and period prevalence*

$$\text{Point prevalence} = \frac{\text{Number of persons ill at a time point}}{\text{Total number in the group at a time point}}$$

$$\text{Period prevalence} = \frac{\text{Number of persons ill during a time period}}{\text{Average size of population during a time period}}$$

B. *Incidence proportion and incidence rate*

$$\text{Incidence proportion} = \frac{\text{Number of new cases}}{\text{Total population at risk}} \times \text{Multiplier (e.g. 100,000)}$$

Note: the multiplier is used simply to avoid fractions and then the incidence is expressed as a figure per multiplier value (for example, incidence per 100,000).

$$\text{Incidence rate} = \frac{\text{Number of new cases during the time period}}{\text{Total person-time of observation}}$$

Note: person-time is usually measured in person-years.

---

prevalence represents the proportion of the population recorded as having the disease over a specified time period. *Incidence cases* are the number of new cases that come into being in a specified population during a specified period of time. Two measures based on incidence cases are usually calculated (Box 3.1B). The **incidence proportion (or cumulative incidence)** is the proportion of unaffected individuals who, on average, will contract the disease of interest over a specified period of time. The **incidence rate** (IR) (also called **incidence density**) measures the rapidity with which newly diagnosed disease develops. To estimate the incidence rate, one observes a population, counts the number of new cases of disease in that population and measures the net time that people are at risk (called person-time and usually measured in person-years).

Making comparisons

To make comparisons between sets of continuous data, the researcher has to ensure that the measurements are defined in exactly the same way. This may involve standardizing to refer to a common base or denominator or may involve ensuring that the definition used in the numerator is consistent. For example, it is of little use to compare the raw mortality counts in, say, one industrial sector with those generated in another if they have very large differences in their workforce size. Some transformation of these raw figures has to occur before valid conclusions relating to the frequency of health problems in each of these sectors can be made. Usually, in epidemiology, this **standardization** can take three forms:

● A *crude rate* is that presented for an entire population.
● A *specific rate* is presented for a particular subgroup of a population (for example, age groups or women versus men). An age-specific mortality rate is simply the mortality rate for a particular age group.
● *Standardized* or *adjusted ratios* are used to compare two or more populations controlling for the effects of age or other variables. An area with a young population, for example, is expected to have a lower crude death rate than one with an old population. We need to compare effects but with the influence of age removed, and hence we need to generate a standardized rate.

To illustrate standardization, consider the case of mortality measurement. Box 3.2 draws on a comparative analysis of mortality in Newcastle-upon-Tyne, England, and Dar Es Salaam, Tanzania. It is drawn from Unwin *et al.* (1997). The crude mortality rates imply that Dar Es Salaam has a

---

Box 3.2 Death rates and specific death rates

	Total deaths A	Mid-year population B	Crude death rate per 1000 population per year (A/B) × 1000
Newcastle	3558	259,541	13.71
Dar Es Salaam	576	66,085	8.72

Age group	Age-specific mortality rate (Deaths per 1000 population per year)	
	Newcastle	Dar Es Salaam
0–4	2.9	18.6
5–14	0.3	2.9
15–24	0.4	2.6
25–34	0.9	7.9
35–44	1.7	8.9
45–54	5.6	12.2
55–64	13.5	30.2
65–74	36.8	55.1
75–84	75.4	105.8
85+	173.8	174.9

Source: Unwin *et al.* 1997.

healthier population. However, in every age group, the age-specific mortality rates are higher in Dar Es Salaam. The reason for this is the existence of different age structures between the two places. In Dar Es Salaam, more people are young. At the very least therefore, we need to take into account the age structures of the two populations. One way to do this is to compare the age-specific death rates, but the method becomes rather cumbersome when comparing many age groups. An alternative and more efficient method is to calculate a single rate that *adjusts* for the age difference between populations.

Two methods of standardization can be employed (Box 3.3). With *direct standardization*, the proportions in each age group of a standard population (for example, the world population; the European population; a national population) are applied to the age-specific death rates of the populations being compared. The same principle is used with *indirect standardization* but here a standard population is used to provide age-specific death rates rather than the proportions of the population in different age groups. This results in an *expected* number of deaths based on applying the age-specific death rates of a standard population to each of the populations being compared. The ratio of the actual (or observed) deaths to the expected deaths is then calculated. This is termed the **standardized mortality ratio** (SMR) and is frequently used in epidemiological studies to compare death rates between different population groups.

If the SMR is equal to 100, then the standard population and study population have the same mortality experience. The observed number of deaths is the same as that expected. If the SMR is greater than 100, then the study population's mortality experience is higher than that of the standard population. If it is less than 100, then the study population's mortality is lower than that of the standard population. Box 3.3B illustrates the indirect calculation of the SMR for Newcastle using the age-specific death rates for England and Wales as the base standard. The 'expected' column is calculated by multiplying the number of people in each age group in Newcastle by the death rate for that age group. The final figure representing the SMR is calculated using the ratio of the total number of actual deaths (given as 3558 in Box 3.2) to the total number of expected deaths. This final SMR figure of 114 tells us that Newcastle's mortality experience is 14 per cent higher than that of England and Wales as a whole. A value below 100 would indicate a favourable experience.

There are a number of problems with age-standardized rates. First, with the direct method, it is necessary to have the age-specific death rates for the population in question. Whilst these are often published (or can be calculated) for country level, they are not so readily available on a city or regional scale. Secondly, the indirect standardized mortality ratio is a comparison between a study population and a standard population. Different study populations' SMRs are not strictly comparable unless the age-mortality relationship between the study population and the reference population is likely to be the same. SMRs are, however, often used in this way to compare the mortality experience of different geographical areas, social classes and other population groups such as those based on sex and ethnicity.

Box 3.3 Direct and indirect standardization

A. *Direct standardization*

Age group	Proportion of standard population in each age group	Newcastle Age-specific death rate multiplied by proportion in standard population	Dar Es Salaam Age-specific death rate multiplied by proportion in standard population
0–4	0.07	0.21	1.30
5–14	0.10	0.03	0.35
15–24	0.14	0.05	0.36
25–34	0.16	0.15	1.26
35–44	0.14	0.24	1.24
45–54	0.12	0.68	1.47
55–64	0.10	1.35	3.02
65–74	0.09	3.31	4.96
75–84	0.06	4.52	6.35
85+	0.02	3.48	3.50
Total	**1.00**	**14.02**	**23.81**

Thus the directly age-adjusted rate for Newcastle is 14.02 deaths per 1000 population per year and for Dar Es Salaam is 23.81 deaths per 1000 population per year.

B. *Indirect standardization*

Age group	Age-specific death rates (per 1000 population) for England and Wales in 1991 A	Number of people ('000) in Newcastle in 1991 by age group B	Expected number of deaths A × B
0–4	1.79	17.030	30
5–14	0.19	30.667	6
15–24	0.57	36.574	21
25–34	0.68	41.786	28
35–44	1.40	34.128	48
45–54	3.70	26.655	99
55–64	10.94	27.345	299
65–74	29.10	25.407	739
75–84	71.46	15.552	1111
85+	166.44	4.397	732
Total		259.541	3113

$$\text{SMR} = \frac{\text{Observed number of deaths}}{\text{Expected number of deaths}} \times 100 = \frac{3558}{3113} \times 100 = 114$$

The indirect method is the more popular approach for two main reasons. First, it is not necessary to know the age-specific death rates of the study population – only the total number of deaths and the age structure are required. Secondly, the method is less prone to errors associated with small numbers because only the total number of observed deaths is used not the number in each specific group. The number of deaths, for example, in the young age groups will be very small and will have large sampling fluctuations.

In the example, the SMR has been standardized for age alone. It is well documented, however, that there are significant sex differences in mortality experience and, very often, age and sex standardized SMRs are calculated. Here, expected values would be calculated by applying the *sex-specific* death rates for each age group as they exist in the standard population (in this case England and Wales) to the number of males and females in each age group for the study population (in this case Newcastle).

Statistical inference

After calculating SMRs as shown above, or indeed any other epidemiological measure, the researcher needs to be able to make a judgement regarding the reliability of the findings. To do this, it is necessary to recognize that, if the age categories had been altered slightly then the end result would have been different. Futhermore, the data will also experience random fluctuations and the researcher will need to assess whether the calculated statistic is due to chance. Most importantly, the researcher needs to know if the value is worth worrying about. In the case of SMRs, for example, the researcher would want to know, given the impact of these challenges to reliability, the range within which there can be confidence that the true SMR lies. The researcher will also want to be certain that the calculated value is significantly different from 100. **Inference** and, specifically, inferential statistical methods help the researcher to make these judgements. There are many research textbooks that document and exemplify scores of commonly used inferential tests. Different tests exist for different types of data and different research designs. The concepts and ideas behind them are consistent across all inferential methods and are summarized in the appendix to this book. Bryman and Cramer (1994, 1996) provide instructions on how to carry out many tests using SPSS and Minitab statistical software. Here, the methods will be illustrated by testing the **significance** of an SMR and generating a **confidence interval** for the value (Box 3.4).

Case study: Ischaemic heart disease

The key features of cross-sectional epidemiology are well illustrated by the example of ischaemic heart disease (IHD), also known as coronary heart disease (CHD). This disease is caused by the reduction or complete obstruction of the flow of blood through the coronary arteries (DoH 1998a).

Box 3.4 Inference and SMRs

A. *Testing an SMR for significance*

Using our earlier example, the researcher needs to determine whether the SMR for Newcastle (114) differs sufficiently from 100 to be classed as a significant value and not one generated by chance.
   An indicator of this chance element can be given by:

$$\text{Indicator} = \frac{(O - E)^2}{E}$$

where O = observed number of deaths and E represents the expected number. In this instance the result is:

$$\frac{(3558 - 3113)^2}{3113} = 63.61$$

The indicator calculated here is known as the chi-square value (χ^2) and the larger the value, the greater the difference between the observed and the expected values. If the χ^2 value in this type of test exceeds 3.8, then the value would be accepted as significant. This is because a value greater than this would only be expected to occur through chance 5 times out of 100 (i.e. with a probability of less than 0.5). The value (3.8) is therefore the *critical* value when the probability p is less than 0.05, i.e. $p < 0.05$. Here the calculated value is 63.61 and therefore large; the researcher would conclude that this difference is not due to a chance element and Newcastle indeed has an SMR which is well above the national average.

B. *Identifying the confidence interval for an SMR*

How confident can we be that the Newcastle SMR is indeed 114? What is the *credible* interval around the given value that is supported by the data? To calculate this we need to know what spread (standard error – see Appendix) we might expect with the Newcastle data. This is given as:

$$\frac{\text{SMR}}{\sqrt{\text{Expected}}} = \frac{114}{\sqrt{3113}} = \frac{114}{55.79} = 2.04$$

A 95% confidence interval can then be calculated as follows:

SMR ± 1.96(2.04)

For the Newcastle data this gives upper limits of 114 + (1.96 × 2.04) = 118, and lower limits of 114 − (1.96 × 2.04) = 110.
   In other words, this means that, given the observed SMR and the expected number of deaths based on a national death rate, the researcher can be confident that, 95 times out of 100, the real value of the Newcastle SMR will lie in the range 110–118. Because the range does not overlap 100 (the 'national average mortality'), the researcher can also be sure that Newcastle has an above-average SMR.

It results from a narrowing of the heart arteries caused by the build-up of fatty deposits in the walls of the heart arteries (atherosclerosis) or by a blood clot (thrombosis). IHD, if not properly managed, can lead to chest pain (angina pectoris), heart attack (acute myocardial infarction), irregular heart beat (arrhythmia) and heart failure. The disease process, once established, is largely irreversible, hence preventive measures are considered to be the most effective means of decreasing the incidence of IHD (Langham *et al.* 1994).

IHD is an important disease to consider, as the burden of the disease to both individuals and society is considerable. In 1995, cardiovascular diseases accounted for almost 15 million deaths worldwide and represented almost 30 per cent of all deaths (WHO 1995). Although mortality rates from IHD have declined in the West since the 1970s, in the UK, IHD remains the biggest single cause of death (ONS 1998). The disease leads to reduced quality of life, can affect ability to work, and is a major cause of premature death. It has been estimated that IHD accounts for 2.4 per cent of NHS hospital expenditure and 1.8 per cent of NHS primary care expenditure (NHSE 1996a). Diseases of the circulatory system, of which IHD is the most common, cost the NHS and personal social services approximately £3.8 billion each year and account for 35 million lost working days (DoH 1998a). In the UK, heart disease, together with strokes, has been identified as one of four national priority areas for action. The consultation paper *Our Healthier Nation* (DoH 1998b) set a national target of reducing the death rate from heart disease, stroke and related illnesses amongst people under the age of 65 by at least one-third by the year 2010.

Morbidity data in theory provide a more complete description of the extent of disease in the population than mortality data. However, as discussed in the previous chapter, there are significant difficulties inherent in collecting morbidity data. Most routine morbidity data collection systems are dependent upon patients recognizing symptoms and subsequently presenting to a health care professional. This is unlikely to provide an accurate picture of the actual incidence/prevalence of IHD as many sufferers will not recognize early symptoms or not present for care. There may additionally be variation in the detection rates of conditions between practitioners and over time. Nevertheless, some idea of the level of IHD can be obtained through the survey of Morbidity Statistics from General Practice (MSGP). This survey reports on the rates of patients consulting with general practitioners. The survey has been subject to criticism owing to the limited sample base used and the self-selecting nature of the 'sentinel' practices that volunteer to take part (OPCS 1995). However, the latest data from this survey show that consulting rates for IHD increase with age and that for all ages the rates are higher for males than for females (Figure 3.3). In addition to the findings of the MSGP survey, hospital activity data and information from the prescription pricing authority can also be used to estimate the levels of IHD in the community. Cross-sectional surveys have largely substantiated the general picture of IHD morbidity emerging from routine sources. The British Regional Heart Survey (Shaper *et al.* 1984) found that nearly one-quarter of middle-aged men showed some evidence of heart disease.

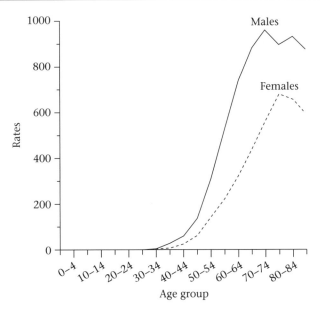

Figure 3.3 Male and female ischaemic heart disease rates (per 100, 000 population) by age.
Source: OPCS 1995: 46.

Variations in distribution of IHD

Time

Long-term trends in mortality have enabled the identification of a number of transitions in health. The phases of transition reflect developments in living conditions, lifestyles and the effectiveness of health interventions. The early part of this century has seen a marked decline in the proportion of deaths from infectious diseases. By the 1960s, diseases of the cardiovascular system, of which IHD is a major component, were the largest cause of death. Since the 1980s, however, European countries have seen a decline in the prominence of cardiovascular deaths and the emergence of cancers as the primary cause of death (Caselli 1994).

From the mid-1950s to the mid-1960s, mortality rates for IHD for males aged under 65 in England and Wales rose, whilst those in older age groups fell. The net result of this was little overall change in the mortality rate due to IHD (Figure 3.4). Since the 1980s there have been sharp falls in IHD mortality rate in younger age groups and a small decline in that for older age groups leading to fall in the all-ages rate. For females, a sharp decrease in mortality rates in older age groups can be seen during the 1950s. More recently the pattern for females is similar to that for males, with greater decreases in rates in younger age groups.

Place

Considerable differences have been observed in mortality rates from cardiovascular diseases in general, and IHD in particular. Cardiovascular diseases

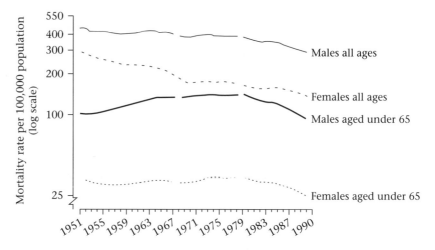

Figure 3.4 Male and female coronary heart disease over time.
Source: DoH 1994: 18.

in general are diseases of the developed world. There are also substantial differences in IHD mortality between the developed nations, with the lowest rates occurring in Japan. Within Europe, mortality rates tend to be lower in the Mediterranean countries, and range from 260 per 100,000 population in Ireland to 67 per 100,000 in France (1988 data) (Puska 1990; DoH 1994).

In England and Wales, place-based variations in IHD mortality rates have been noted in a number of studies (Mohan *et al.* 1990; Curtis *et al.* 1993). Recent data (Figure 3.5) confirm a pattern of relatively high mortality rates from IHD in the north of England and in Wales, and generally lower rates in south east England. This geographical pattern has been found since the 1920s (Britton 1990). Indeed, whilst time trends at the national level show decreasing levels of mortality from IHD, this overall decrease has been accompanied by widening inequalities between the most and the least deprived areas within England and Wales (Bryce *et al.* 1994). Addressing such *spatial* inequalities has become an important element of recent UK policy (DoH 1995, 1998b, 1999).

Person

There is a clear trend of rising IHD mortality and morbidity with age. There are also significant differences between the sexes. At younger ages mortality from IHD and prevalence, as shown by the MSGP data, are much greater in males than in females. The difference is much reduced in postmenopausal women. This observed variation has led to the hypothesis that oestrogen is protective against IHD (Wenger 1997). Nevertheless, there has until recently been a disproportionate amount of research interest in IHD in males (Thomas 1998) and some evidence that women are less likely than men to be diagnosed and receive appropriate treatment for IHD (Clarke *et al.* 1994; Wenger 1997).

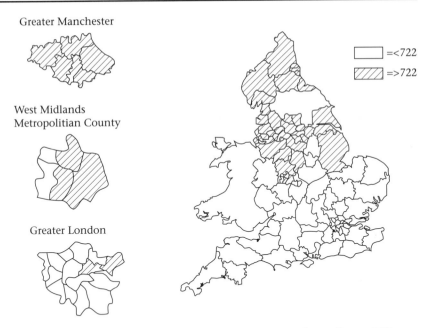

Figure 3.5 Mortality rates (per 100, 000) from coronary heart disease (ICD 410–414) in persons aged 65–74 by Health Authority (April 1996 boundaries), 1993 to 1995.
Source: Adapted from DoH/NIE (1996)

Table 3.1 Ethnic variation in coronary heart disease

	Men		Women	
Country of birth	*No. of deaths*	*SMR (95% CI)*	*No. of deaths*	*SMR (95% CI)*
Total population	123,741	100	44,110	100
Scotland	3,066	120 (116–124)	1,099	130 (122–137)
Ireland	3,995	124 (120–127)	1,398	120 (114–126)
East Africa	372	131 (118–145)	73	105 (82–132)
West Africa	81	56 (44–70)	16	62 (35–100)
Caribbean	592	46 (42–49)	236	71 (61–80)
South Asia	3,348	146 (141–151)	882	151 (141–162)

CI = confidence interval
Source: Wild and McKeigue 1997.

Routine mortality data have identified significant differences in mortality from IHD between different ethnic groups. In England and Wales, mortality from IHD has been found to be low in Caribbean immigrants and high in South Asian immigrants (Table 3.1) when compared with the national average (Balarajan 1991). Furthermore, these differences in IHD mortality have widened between 1970 and 1992 and are thought not to be attributable to variations in the socioeconomic backgrounds of the different populations (Wild and McKeigue 1997).

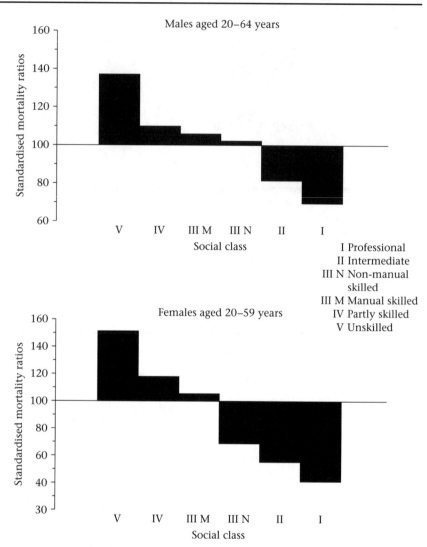

Figure 3.6 Social class and coronary heart disease.
Source: DoH 1995: 104.

The Black Report (DHSS 1980), and more recently the Acheson Inquiry into health inequalities (Acheson 1998), have highlighted an association between poor health and social class. Variation in IHD mortality conforms to this finding. Mortality arising from IHD shows a gradient of increasing standardized mortality ratios, rising from less than the national average for social class I to greater than the national average for social class V (the lowest social class) (Figure 3.6). The variation with respect to social class is similar for both sexes.

Table 3.2 Risk factors for coronary heart disease

Major established factors [a]	Less established factors [b]
Individual	
Sex	High density lipoprotein cholesterol
Age	Other lipids
Blood pressure	Glucose intolerance, insulin levels
Serum (plasma) cholesterol	Obesity
Cigarette smoking	Physical activity
	Psychosocial factors
	Social class
	Social mobility
	Ethnic group
	Personality type
	Familial factors
	Contraceptive pill
	Clotting factors and fibrinolysis
	Diet
Group	
Diet	Water hardness

[a] Consistently shown to be powerful factors in many different studies over many years.
[b] Inconsistent, less powerful, less commonly or more recently investigated, or factors in which epidemiological techniques are poorly developed.
Source: Farmer *et al.* 1996: 112.

Risk factors

Investigation of the risk factors associated with IHD was directed by the findings of early descriptive studies. The hypotheses generated by these descriptive cross-sectional studies led to a number of landmark analytical studies (largely cohort studies – see Chapter 5). These later studies sought to build upon the descriptive work and confirm hypothesized risk factors for IHD. Among these analytical studies were the Framingham Heart Study and the Tecumseh study in the USA, and the British Regional Heart Study.

Table 3.2 identifies a range of risk factors for IHD. Subsequent research has provided evidence that identifies high-density lipoprotein cholesterol as an additional established risk factor (ONS 1997b). The established risk factors identified above are investigated regularly using the Health Survey for England. Informants are classified as having IHD if they report ever having a heart attack or angina which has been confirmed by a doctor. In addition to these self-reported measures, the survey uses the Rose Angina Questionnaire (Rose *et al.* 1977) to provide back-up prevalence estimates.

The 1994 HSE found that higher levels of blood pressure, cholesterol and smoking in both males and females were associated with a higher prevalence of IHD. This is called a *positive association*. There was an inverse relationship between prevalence of IHD in men and women and levels of physical activity. Prevalence is highest in those who exercise least; this may also be referred to as a *negative association*. The HSE also found that, whilst ex-drinkers had the highest prevalence of IHD, non-drinkers had a higher prevalence than moderate current drinkers. This supports the hypothesis of a U-shaped curve to the health-damaging effects of alcohol, with moderate levels of alcohol consumption conferring a protective effect when compared with abstinence and excessive consumption (Marmot and Brunner 1991).

The HSE provides valuable information on the prevalence of combinations of risk factors for IHD. Amongst those surveyed who were found to be on treatment for high blood pressure, 21 per cent of men drank more than 21 units of alcohol per week and 8 per cent of women drank more than 14 units per week. These levels of drinking are the nationally accepted thresholds above which alcohol consumption is defined as health-damaging. Almost one in five of men and women with a previous history of cardiovascular disease (defined as angina, heart attack or stroke) were found to continue to smoke. Forty-two per cent of men and 57 per cent of women with high blood pressure were found to have a high cholesterol level. Of those with a past history of cardiovascular disease, 16 per cent of men and 18 per cent of women were found to have high blood pressure at the time of the survey but were not receiving any medication to lower their blood pressure. The inclusion of geographical data in the survey also allows analysis of multiple risks. Compared with the country as a whole, men with high blood pressure in the north of England (where IHD rates are higher) were significantly more likely to drink over 21 units of alcohol per week.

Impact on policy

National and regional differences in IHD rates identified through descriptive epidemiological studies have provided a valuable starting point for identifying risks. The subsequent confirmation of these risks using the analytical methods covered in the next two chapters provides a focus for primary prevention measures.

In 1974 the WHO initiated the Comprehensive Cardiovascular Community Control Programme (CCCCP) in Europe (Puska 1990). This programme combined medical and epidemiological knowledge to identify risk factors that were to become the focus of community and public health based approaches to modifying the risk profile of the population. This strategy was deliberately broad and ran counter to the more normal approach of aiming interventions at those at high risk. From the epidemiological perspective, the approach acknowledged that major reductions in IHD rates could only be achieved by a widespread reduction in the levels of known risk factors and that this required community-wide action. The risk factors identified were smoking, high serum cholesterol levels, high blood pressure, physical inactivity, overweight and excess alcohol consumption.

Such a community programme approach is also reflected in UK policy developments. The promotion of 'heart health' using interventions based on epidemiological evidence is an important element of the *Health of the Nation* strategy (DoH 1992) and more recently *Our Healthier Nation* (DoH 1998b, 1999). Whilst these strategies identify primary prevention at the population level as being central to the reduction of IHD they also recognize that specific high-risk groups provide an opportunity for targeted preventative programmes.

Conclusion

Descriptive epidemiological techniques including cross-sectional surveys provide an valuable set of tools for identifying areas of need, for quantifying those with a need and for monitoring progress towards reducing the morbidity and mortality burdens of disease. This chapter has also highlighted the importance of these techniques in generating hypotheses about possible causes of ill health.

Summary

- Cross-sectional studies, also known as prevalence studies, are a particular type of descriptive study. Cross-sectional studies are useful when a snapshot of disease prevalence is required.

- An important variant of the basic cross-sectional study is the repeated cross-sectional study. The Health Survey for England (HSE) is an example of a repeated cross-sectional study.

- Epidemiological surveys will often involve the collection of background information about respondents. Some of this information will be continuous in nature. There are many tools for continuous data description and analysis. These include both graphical techniques and statistical tests.

- To make comparisons between sets of continuous data, the researcher has to ensure that the measurements are defined in exactly the same way. This may involve standardizing to refer to a common base. The standardization of mortality data provides a case example.

- Researchers also need to be able to make judgements regarding the reliability of their findings. This involves use of the statistical concept 'confidence'.

- The hypotheses generated by descriptive cross-sectional studies often lead on to analytical studies.

Further reading

On basic descriptive data analysis, see:

Marsh, C. (1988) *Exploring Data*. Cambridge: Polity Press.

For further detail on cross-sectional studies, review the relevant material in other books on epidemiology, for example:

Hennekens, C. and Buring, J. (1987) *Epidemiology in Medicine*. Boston: Little Brown.
Rothman, K. (1986) *Modern Epidemiology*. Boston: Little Brown.

Unwin, N., Carr, S. and Leeson, J. with Pless-Mulloli, T. (1997) *An Intro-ductory Study Guide to Public Health and Epidemiology.* Buckingham: Open University Press.

Activities

1 Thinking of your own professional area, what are the key prevalence research questions which are currently of interest? Compare your suggested areas of interest with those of your colleagues. Can you think of any reasons why areas of interest might differ?

2 Try to sketch the histograms for the distribution of the following among the adult population: (a) weekly cigarette consumption, (b) shoe size, (c) height, (d) age at death. Indicate which are normally distributed, positively skewed or negatively skewed.

3 Using the indirect method, calculate and interpret the standardized mortality ratio (SMR) for a place with 1223 deaths using the following information:

Age (years)	Local population ('000)	National death rate (per 1000)
0–1	0.74	19.78
1–4	2.93	0.76
5–14	8.38	0.40
15–24	8.83	0.92
25–44	13.41	1.62
45–64	18.36	13.45
65–74	8.23	51.82
75+	4.64	137.42

4 Referring back to Box 3.4, remember that the χ^2 calculation takes into account the observed number of deaths. Assume that the same SMR had been generated with a smaller number of deaths – 3200 observed deaths and 2807 expected. What would be the χ^2 for this SMR? Calculate the confidence interval as well and comment on both results.

PRINCIPLES AND EXPERIMENTS

In this chapter we begin our discussion of some of the more complex ways in which epidemiologists go about their work. In particular, we consider in more detail the matter of epidemiological **study design**: recipes for conducting research and gaining information about the health of people and the causes of disease. Epidemiologists recognize a number of types of design that differ in terms of effectiveness – how well they do the job – and efficiency – how cheaply or quickly they do it. The choice of a particular design depends on the purpose and requirements of the research. The overall objective is to obtain accurate and precise results with limited resources.

After completing this chapter you should be able to:

● discuss the key principles underpinning analytical epidemiological designs;
● assess the relative strengths and weaknesses of experimental design in epidemiology.

Our overall aim is to turn you into informed, critical appraisers of epidemiological research. Even in published literature, misleading results can get through the scrutiny of referees, and no journal offers a guarantee as to the validity of its papers. It is therefore vital to be able to assess whether the conclusions of a study are valid and to understand the limitations of such studies.

We begin by considering what we mean by causation and then discuss the general problems facing researchers in collecting reliable information that will lead to valid conclusions. Attention then turns to an assessment

of the randomized clinical trial, the most robust of the study designs
employed in epidemiological research.

Causation and causality

As we have already found out, the purpose of an epidemiological study
may be to describe the occurrence of disease (*descriptive epidemiology*), and
to explore the causation of disease (*aetiological or analytical epidemiology*).
The latter aims to explore disease causation by evaluating the effect of an
'exposure' on the risk of developing disease. A researcher might thus
enquire whether air pollution causes bronchitis or whether a particular
chemical causes lung cancer. In such situations, epidemiologists frequently
imply causal explanations by using such phrases as 'results in', 'accounts
for', 'influenced by' and even 'explained by'.

Epidemiologists hold a particular causal view of the world. This can be
best described as multicausal. With multicausality, each effect has a number
of causes and each cause can produce a number of effects. For example,
consider the causal relationships in Figure 4.1 in which a single-headed
arrow signifies a possible causal relationship from cause to effect. Here there
are multiple causes and multiple effects; and effects in one causal model
can be causes in another. This complex patterning of causes and effects is
known as a web of causation or a multifactorial aetiology (MacMahon
and Pugh 1970).

In this multicausal world no effect is *sufficient* in its own right in that
the operation of the causal factor always results in disease. Nor is any
effect *necessary* in its own right; it is possible to get the disease without
having received a particular exposure. Thus, not all regular smokers get
lung cancer, and there are people with lung cancer who have never smoked.
This means we also have to deal with a probabilistic version of causality.
We are interested in whether cigarette smoking leads to an increased *risk*
of getting lung cancer. Epidemiologists pay a great deal of attention to the
accurate quantitative assessment of this risk.

How do we know if an observed association is causal or not? Following
a long tradition going back to J.S. Mill (1806–73) we can recognize three
conditions for a causal relationship. If they are all met, then the relationship is deemed causal. If any one of them is not met then the relationship
is not causal. The first condition is that of **co-variation**. Exposure and
disease should co-vary over space and time. If air pollution is a cause of
bronchitis then an increase in air pollution should be associated with an
increase in bronchitis and highly polluted parts of the country should
have a high incidence of bronchitis. If an increase in the exposure produces an increase in the disease, there is a *positive* causal relationship; if
an increase in the exposure produces a decrease in disease, the relationship is a *negative* one, and the exposure is seen as protective. This aspect
of causality requires valid measures of exposure and disease and a means
of assessing the degree and nature of the association.

Temporal precedence is the second criterion. This simply means that, to
be causal, changes in exposure must come before and not after changes in

disease state. This seemingly obvious statement – that a cause must precede its effect – is far from straightforward in the real world. The identification of temporal precedence is often plagued by time lags (a long latent period between the exposure and the disease) and possible reciprocal causation. For example, a person may be caused to be depressed by losing a job, or the loss of a job may be caused by the inability to work effectively owing to depression. If we are going to be clear about this aspect of causality we are going to need observations over time and preferably observations that follow the same individuals.

The third and final condition is that other possible explanations of the cause and effect have been eliminated. The researcher seeks other 'hidden' or 'lurking' variables that are causally prior to both the exposure and the outcome, and which are really producing the apparent association. For example, is it smoking that kills workers, or is it working in a high-risk environment that kills smokers? To deal with this aspect of causality we need to be able to **control** or 'allow for' these third variables.

Threats to validity

Epidemiologists are particularly concerned to ensure the validity of their studies. There are two broad types of validity. **External validity** refers to the extent to which the results of a study can be generalized to a wider population. In some cases, the problems are easy to see. Can chemicals that are found to be non-toxic on animals be safely given to people, or are the results species specific? More subtly, can results derived from one occupational group, such as doctors or bus drivers, be transferred to all occupational groups. **Internal validity** concerns the results within a study, and in particular how easily an association between exposure and outcome can be found due to non-causal reasons. Three general factors are recognized as reducing the internal validity of a study: *bias* (systematic error), **confounding** (an unrecognized variable influencing the observed results) and *random error* (chance).

Both internal and external validity are important but it is internal validity that is of primary importance. Studies that have high internal validity always have some value, even if the external validity is low. A study with low internal validity is worthless. It is useful at this point to get a preliminary understanding of the issues involved by examining each of the possible causes of internal invalidity.

Bias

As previously discussed, the main purpose of an aetiological study is to estimate the effect of an exposure on the risk of developing a disease. Bias may arise in two main ways. **Selection bias** occurs when subjects who are selected and participate in a study are different in a systematic way from those excluded from the study. Obviously we cannot study everybody in a population and we have to have some way of selecting them. Under optimal circumstances, the method for inclusion of subjects leads to a valid comparison between the exposed and the unexposed that, in turn, yields correct information regarding a disease risk. The selection process itself, however, may distort the exposure–disease relationship. Thus, whenever a survey has a low response rate there is a danger of selection bias, because the non-responders may be atypical, or differ from the responders in some systematic way. Similarly, if a study has a high loss of respondents as they are followed over time (**attrition**), there is a cause for concern because it may be that people with particular characteristics are dropping out of the study. Many investigators believe that high participation rates are crucial to the validity of epidemiological findings.

Information bias is the systematic gap between the measured value and true value of either the exposure or the disease. Much of epidemiology uses categorizations, and information bias can occur when people are systematically misclassified. Disease misclassification is when a person with a disease is incorrectly labelled as healthy and vice versa. Exposure misclassification is when a person who has been exposed is regarded as being unexposed and vice versa. There are many sources of this sort of bias, including faulty measuring instruments, varying standards in different laboratories, mistakes in data management, and misreporting of symptoms by subjects trying to please the investigator. Some forms of this bias are given specific names. **Recall bias** refers to situations where those with the disease are more likely to recall past exposures, such as when mothers with deformed babies recall more accurately the number of times they were exposed to X-rays during pregnancy. *Interviewer bias* is where awareness of the presence or absence of disease in a subject may influence the interviewer in his or her recording of exposures. With *unacceptability bias*, subjects may reply to a question about exposure with a socially acceptable but sometimes inaccurate response. For example, people tend to underestimate their alcohol consumption.

No study is immune from the possibility of bias. The researcher must therefore consider potential sources of bias when selecting subjects, collecting information, analysing results and interpreting findings. With planning it is possible to anticipate and avoid certain types of error and thus conduct a study that leads to a convincing and valid conclusion. Indeed, if this cannot be achieved, it might be better to refrain from doing the study at all. No end of analysis will rescue biased results. In published studies you should critically evaluate how the study groups were selected, how the information about exposure and disease was collected, and how the data were analysed. Box 4.1 summarizes some general guidelines for combating the possibility of bias in epidemiological studies.

Confounding

The second threat to validity is confounding. Let us examine this issue using an example drawn from Jones and Moon (1987). It may be suggested that overcrowding causes bronchitis. Such an association can occur for one of three reasons: there may be a true causal relationship, the association may occur simply by chance, or the true cause may be some

> **Box 4.1 Preventing bias**
>
> *To prevent selection bias:*
>
> - Develop an explicit definition of what constitutes a case of a disease, and what constitutes an exposure.
> - Aim for high participation rates.
> - Take precautions to ensure representativeness and try to check for this.
>
> *To prevent measurement bias:*
>
> - Validate exposures by using more than one source of information.
> - If possible, ensure that interviewers do not know the subjects' disease status.
> - Provide standardized training sessions and protocols for interviewers.
> - Use standardized data collection forms.
> - Try to ensure complete data are collected on all subjects in a uniform manner.

third variable, air pollution. It is possible to recognize three fundamentally different types of relationship between the variables (Figure 4.1). First, there is the possibility that living at high densities and suffering air pollution are both independent causes of bronchitis. If such a relationship exists, the lowering of overcrowding and air pollution levels would result in lower death rates, the lowest rates occurring when both crowding and air pollution are reduced. The alternative model is one where only air pollution is truly a cause of bronchitis. The original association between overcrowding and bronchitis is a *spurious* one produced by the association of air pollution and overcrowding. Subareas of a city may have both high air pollution and a great deal of overcrowding, but it may be only the former variable that is causally linked to chest disease. If overcrowding is reduced, but air pollution remains at previous levels, this model suggests that bronchitis deaths would not decrease.

Confounding is therefore a process whereby the association between exposure and outcome is distorted by the association between the confounder and both the exposure and outcome. A factor is therefore a confounding factor only when the two associations exist: when the factor is associated with both the exposure and the outcome under assessment. It is important to stress that there can be relationships between variables that do not constitute confounding. Continuing the bronchitis example, we can suggest the third model, which is known as a causal chain. In this example, air pollution plays the role of an *intervening* variable that is on the causal path between a determinant and an outcome. High-density living produces high air pollution which in turn produces bronchitis. Confounding is not introduced by a factor that is simply an intermediate step in the causal path between exposure and disease.

We can take the issue of confounding a step further if we turn to the example of smoking and lung cancer. For many people, the simple causal

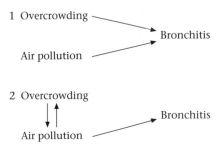

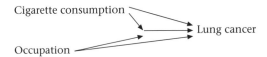

3 Overcrowding ⟶ Air pollution ⟶ Bronchitis

Figure 4.1   Three causal relationships.

Cigarette consumption ⟶ Lung cancer
Occupation ⟶

Figure 4.2   Synergistic interaction and effect modification.

relationship that cigarette consumption leads to lung cancer is undisputed. While the majority of researchers believe in the essential validity of this model, others, however, continue to argue that alternative models are more appropriate. Doll and Peto (1981) have estimated that smoking accounts for some 30 per cent of all cancers, occupational factors cause less than 5 per cent of all cancers and pollution only 2 per cent. Epstein (1979) argues to the contrary that occupational carcinogens produce anything between 20 and 40 per cent of all cancers and the contribution of smoking has been overestimated. Epstein's fundamental model is that there is a **synergistic interaction** between smoking and occupation (Figure 4.2). In this model, both smoking and occupation are independent causes of cancer, but they also interact: the people most likely to develop cancer work in a carcinogenic environment and are smokers. According to this view, occupation is not a confounder but modifies the effect of the smoking exposure variable. The term **effect modifier** is used for such a variable.

Any relationship between two variables (be it positive or negative, weak, strong or non-existent) should not be taken at face value. Techniques are required to control for potential confounders or 'third' variables. In essence there are two distinct approaches to this task: control is achieved either *by design* before the data are collected, or *by analysis* after data collection. In terms of design, we will see in subsequent discussion that confounding can be dealt with by *restricting* the participation in the study to certain individuals, *matching* individuals with others, and by a process known as **randomization**. In the analysis phase we can *restrict* analysis to certain types of individual; we may divide or *stratify* the data into subgroups by categories of the confounding factor, or we may use **multivariate analysis** to take into account the effect of more than one factor simultaneously. Often, combinations of these different methods are used.

Many studies are open to the charge that the observed differences are in fact due to confounding variables. However, in practice, many potential confounders will not in fact be confounding, in that their associations with outcome and exposure in the study data are often weak and unimportant. But this can only be known if data on the confounders are collected and analysed. In evaluating published research, you should always try to think of any important possible confounders that have not been dealt with.

Random error

The third and final general threat to the credibility of our results is random error. Such error arises due to chance alone; it is purely random, not systematically biased. The term **precision** is used to refer to the degree of absence of random error. Random error is closely related to the degree of inherent *variability* in the measures of both exposure and outcome. It is difficult to appreciate the variability of data about people. Think of lifetime outcomes. We have all heard anecdotes about someone who has smoked 60 cigarettes a day for 60 years without apparent ill effect and the very fit 35-year-old whose sudden death is so shocking. With such variability, observed differences are bound to occur. They may be due to real causal effects, random inherent variation, or both. If we study two identical populations with identical risk factors and exposures, and pick a sample of people for our analyses (say 500 from each), it likely that the disease rates measured will be similar to one another but not identical. As the number of people in our study increases (say to 10,000 subjects each), we expect our study-based estimates of the true disease rates in the entire populations to be more reliable.

The problem of random error is tackled in two ways. First, adjustments can be made to study design. Precision can be improved by increasing either the size of the sample or the duration of follow-up, or both. Put simply, the greater the number of observations, the higher precision. Methods are available to determine how many are needed for reliable results for different types of study design. We do not want a study that has too few observations to give a reliable result (a study that is underpowered). However, it is also important that we do not collect more information than we need in order to produce acceptable results, so cost-efficiency, the relation between precision and cost, is important too. Secondly, we can confront random error at the analysis stage. We can use statistical procedures to derive confidence intervals that describe the degree of uncertainty around any estimate of the degree of association. We can also use statistical tests to come to a decision about whether or not a result is due to chance.

Experimental study designs

Within the broad family of quantitative designs, we can recognize three major groupings:

- **Experimental (or interventionist) designs** in which the invest-igator intervenes to create the desired situation and to manipulate the causal factor to see what effect it has. A key feature of this design is that a process known as randomization is used to determine which subjects are manipulated and which are left alone. Two basic types of randomized design are recognized: *randomized clinical trials* in which the basic unit of intervention is an individual subject, and *community trials* in which the basic unit of intervention is the group.
- *Quasi-experimental designs* which include experiments of opportunity or natural experiments; in such studies the exposure has changed naturally without the direct intervention of the researcher. Quasi-experimental designs are characterized by their lack of randomization.
- *Observational designs* in which the investigator passively observes what is happening in the real world. Events are observed as they happen.

It is observational designs that are the mainstay of epidemiological work and we will devote attention to such designs in the next chapter. An experimental design, the **randomized clinical trial** (RCT) is, however, usually portrayed as the 'gold standard' for epidemiological research. It is seen as the most scientifically rigorous method of hypothesis testing that is available. The particular procedures used in the design are said to guar-antee high validity and watertight conclusions. In practice, while it is widely used to evaluate new treatment and interventions, it is not com-monly used to evaluate the effects of causal agents (except in animal experiments) because of ethical considerations. We will use the remainder of this chapter to discuss the RCT and other interventionist designs so that, by considering the procedures of the 'gold standard', we can later more clearly see the comparative strengths and weaknesses of other designs.

Randomized clinical trials

Consider a laboratory experiment to assess the influence of air pollution in producing lung cancer. A strategy for an RCT might be as follows:

- One hundred male mice aged one week are placed in identical cages, given the same diet and kept at the same temperature. All the mice are X-rayed before the experiments start and any with lung defects are excluded from the experiment.
- Twenty-five of the mice are given pure air; these are the **control group**.
- The remaining 75 mice form the *experimental groups*; they are further divided into three groups of 25, which receive either low, moderate or high doses of polluted air.
- After 15 weeks of such treatment all 100 mice are killed and autopsies are performed. The sizes of any tumours are measured.
- The average size of tumour is plotted against the amount of air pollution.
- If the tumour size increases in a consistent way with pollution there is said to be a *dose–response* relationship. This finding would be highly suggestive that air pollution is *causal* in producing lung cancer. If there is no consistent relationship in the plot of air quality against tumour size, the empirical evidence does not support the pollution–cancer link.

The decision on whether the relationship is causal or not is based on the following key form of argument: *if* we change a possibly causal variable (pollution) *and* keep everything else unchanged (or controlled) *and* observe changes in the outcome variable (lung cancer), *then* these changes must be due to the manipulated variable, that is pollution is the cause of lung cancer.

Four essential elements of experimental design are clearly seen in this protocol. First, the experimenter deliberately intervenes to *manipulate* the amount, timing and frequency of the exposure to air pollution. It is planned that the experimental group receives higher doses than the control group. Here we can note that the experimental design is inherently a *prospective* study, in that experimenters manipulate the cause and only then observe the effect. Knowing exactly when intervention is made ensures temporal precedence, disallows reciprocal causation and often allows the discernment of the latent period as the mice could be measured after any chosen time interval.

Secondly, the study achieves *control*. This takes place by *physical* means (each mouse has been kept at the same temperature), by *standardization* (they are all given identical diets, none had lung defects at the outset) and by *matching* (the mice in the experimental and control groups are of the same age and sex). Control aims to ensure that the control and experimental groups are similar in all respects except for pollution. The use of a control group allows estimation of the natural or background variability of the disease: that amount of lung cancer that occurs without air pollution.

The third element of experimental design is *comparison*. Before the intervention the mice are comparable. There are no essential differences between the mice in the different groups. In our hypothetical study they are very young and will not have been exposed to potential confounding factors. Comparison after the intervention should reveal only the effects of intervention.

Replication is the final issue. It can be seen in this experiment in two senses. It was not just one mouse that was placed in each group but 25 replicates; the larger the number of replicates, the greater the faith we can have in the results (guarding against random error). It is also the case that the protocol for the experiment could be replicated in another laboratory at another time; this should lead to broadly comparable results – if not, there must be an investigation into why this is the case.

Experiments are redolent of the sterilized world of the chemistry laboratory, but the modern experiment was actually developed in the messy world of field research. In the 1920s, R.A. Fisher developed the randomized experiment to evaluate the differential effectiveness of treatments such as manure and fertilizer on crop yields. So far we have ignored this important aspect of experimental design. We have presumed that we know all the factors that have to be controlled, that is we have presumed that there is no confounding. The classical solution to confounding and the need for control in experimental studies was, as we noted above, the use of physical control, standardization and matching. Fisher proposed a brilliant simple alternative solution for dealing with unknown factors, by designing statistical experiments based on the key concept of randomization. With

Table 4.1 The first RCT for the treatment of tuberculosis

			Outcome at 6 months		
			Deaths	Stable or deterioration	Improvement
		52 treated with bed rest alone	14	21	17
107 patients with pulmonary tuberculosis age 15–30 years	Random allocation				
		55 treated with streptomycin and bed rest	4	13	38

Source: data from Medical Research Council 1948.

randomization in our hypothetical example, individual mice would be allocated to particular experimental or control groups by some random device so that every mouse would have an equal probability of being allocated to any one of the groups. For example, if there was only one experimental and one control group, allocation could be decided on the tossing of an unbiased coin, with those mice getting 'heads' receiving the pollution.

While randomization does not place a rigid control over any factor it does mean that we can expect that the average level of all variables (known and unknown, measured or unmeasured) will be approximately the same in both groups. For example, both groups will have roughly the same number of small mice, heavy mice, white mice, and so on. Control has been achieved by design so that the only way in which the two groups will differ is in terms of the experimental variable, pollution. Randomization, in effect, removes confounding and makes other things equal by ensuring similar variability between control and treated subjects due to unmeasured variables. Greater numbers in each group increase our confidence that the groups are equivalent before the experimental changes, and that the observed differences after the experiment are not a result of chance. The incredible achievement of randomization is that it controls all factors simultaneously to a known degree even without knowing what they are.

By the late 1940s Fisher's innovation was being applied to humans. In what we now call randomized clinical trials (RCTs) the experimental group is given a new, untried therapy, drug or vaccine, while the control group is given a treatment in current use or no treatment at all. Randomization, in this context, has the particular advantage that no bias is introduced in the selection of patients in terms of the severity of the disease. Table 4.1 shows what is usually regarded as the earliest example of an RCT. The study started in 1946 and sought to evaluate the effectiveness of a particular chemotherapy (streptomycin) on advanced pulmonary tuberculosis (Medical Research Council 1948).

People are of course different from crops and there is a real problem of achieving control with human populations, with knowing subjects being treated by knowing practitioners. With human beings, the mere fact that they know they are in an experiment may influence the outcome. In clinical trials, patients receiving a treatment that is ineffective are known to show an improvement over the control group receiving no treatment simply because the treated patients are getting care and attention and even hope. This problem can be overcome in the **single-blind experiment** in which the patients do not know whether they are in an experimental group receiving treatment or in a control group receiving an inert treatment known as a **placebo**. Differential attrition bias is also minimized in the single-blind trial by the patients not knowing if they have been assigned to the placebo treatment. The effectiveness of the treatment is then compared with the improvement produced by the placebo. The other feature of the human experiment is that the practitioner delivering the treatment can thwart the design by giving differential care to those on the new treatment or, in the belief that the treatment is going to be effective, giving the new drug to those with the perceived greatest need, thereby thwarting the randomization. This problem is overcome in a **double-blind experiment** where neither the patient not the practitioner knows who has been assigned to which group.

Validity and RCTs

While many researchers believe that experimental research is the most powerful form of scientific investigation, comparatively little human experimental work has been undertaken to investigate disease causation. Undoubtedly, the major reason for this is that it would be unethical to assign persons at random to do things that may cause suffering. For example, imagine taking a healthy group of children aged 10 and forcing half of them to live in overcrowded conditions, to smoke 25 cigarettes a day and to breathe air with high levels of pollution for the next 30 years. Such experiments would not be allowed by the ethical committees that grant permission for experimental research. These committees ensure that researchers adhere to the rule of 'first of all, do no harm'.

A second threat to the validity of RCTs concerns causal relationships of interest that are not amenable to manipulation and random allocation. For example, sex, age, race are fundamentally unalterable. Although they can be controlled through randomization, they cannot be manipulated to gauge causal power. Another difficulty with experimental investigation is that, while the procedures may be internally valid in delivering watertight conclusions, they are poor in terms of external validity. This means that their results do not easily generalize from the artificial experimental situation where potential confounders are the subject of control to a real world where control does not take place and hypothesized relationships are confounded by multiple interactions. With human populations the experimenter may find it difficult to determine whether the treatment would work well in the wider community and under different contexts. For example, restrictive criteria for inclusion of subjects may produce a very homogeneous study population but, at the same time, may restrict the ability to extrapolate results to patients with other characteristics.

Community trials

In RCTs an intervention is specific to individuals. In **community trials**, a group or population is subject to a particular intervention. At its most basic, a community trial is a design which involves at least one intervention site and at least one control site, whether or not randomization is used. Typically the intervention is aimed at everybody in the intervention community, while key outcomes are usually measured at the individual level. There may well be an implicit (and frequently problematic) assumption that individual characteristics are dispersed randomly between the two sites thus providing control.

Community trials (Koepsell 1998a, b) typically aim to evaluate a long-term, large-scale public health intervention for primary prevention, that is prevention before the disease has been caused. This includes studies where the intervention is likely to be community-wide, for example, adding fluoride to drinking water. Community trials are often thus concerned with interventions aimed at the total population not just at those at high risk. Interventions aim to shift the entire distribution of the risk factor downwards and not simply to pull in the top end of those most at risk. For many diseases it is only the minority of cases that occur in high-risk individuals. Community trials therefore have a greater potential for prevention than the targeted strategy.

The community trial approach is usually based on geographical communities. It could, however, be applied to socially defined groups or indeed occupational groups. It can be summarized as a three-stage process:

● Establishing the baseline before intervention, this is usually some measure of disease or exposure incidence or prevalence.
● Making the intervention at the community-wide level.
● Remeasuring the incidence or prevalence to see what change there has been, and comparing the change in the communities that have received the intervention with those that have not.

It may be thought that, with generally a small sample of communities involved in any one study, randomization is optional. This is not the case. Even with small numbers, randomization should be used as it brings (as in RCTs) an element of control over confounders that are unknown or difficult to quantify, and it prevents any suspicion that the investigator has biased the choice of sites for intervention. Consideration should also be given to matching so that, for example, allocation by randomization should be from matched pairs, with the matching done on community characteristics. Thus a high social-class, service-sector community in the intervention group would be matched with a similar community in the control group. The advantages of doing so are potential reductions in bias and gains in precision. However, care must be taken, for if matching is based on a poor correlate of outcome, there may be a loss of power to detect genuine change.

In terms of measuring change, there are in essence two alternatives. First, one might follow a sample of individuals over time and repeatedly measure their behaviour and the outcome; this is a cohort approach and is discussed in more detail in the next chapter. Secondly, it may be possible to conduct two or more surveys in which different people are sampled on each occasion. This is a repeated cross-sectional approach as described in the previous chapter. Cohort samples are ideal for assessing individual-level behavioural change (which is what we are really after), while repeated cross-sectional samples measure changes in prevalence at the community level. The latter may result from a combination of behaviour change and 'turnover' as people migrate into and out of the study communities. However, attrition bias and cost may be high with the cohort approach, and there may be a selection bias in terms of behavioural change for those who are willing to be subjected to repeated measurement. In practice, researchers have often used both cohort and repeated cross-sectional approaches in the same trial.

Consideration should be also be given to collecting not just data on individuals but also on the characteristics of the communities, that is 'community-level indicators'. Cheadle *et al.* (1992) conceptualized several types of community-level measures, which differ according to their obtrusiveness (conspicuousness of the observation process), reactivity (likelihood that measurement itself could lead to changes in outcomes), and unit of observation (such as work sites, restaurants, or the community as a whole). Collecting community-level information is usually substantially less costly than conducting large-scale collection on individuals. There should be no bias owing to inability to blind in making these measurements.

One of the largest examples of a community trial design is the US National Cancer Institute's Community Intervention Trial for Smoking Cessation (COMMIT). This aimed to reduce prevalence of heavy cigarette smoking. In 1986, applications from pairs of communities were invited. Each pair had to be from the same state or province in the USA and Canada, and to be roughly matched in terms of size and demographic make-up. Eleven pairs were chosen and were randomized to control or intervention groups. Each intervention community received an average of $880,000 over four years to fund a public education programme in the media and special events which included activities at community centres and work sites. The effectiveness of the interventions was monitored through a cohort telephone survey of about 1100 smokers in each intervention and control community. Cross-sectional samples of smokers were also surveyed at baseline and after intervention to measure changes in smoking prevalence. The results showed that the quit rate (after adjusting for co-variates) among light to moderate smokers was about three percentage points higher in intervention sites compared with their matched controls. However, no statistically significant differences in quit rates among heavy smokers were found.

The main strength of the community trial is that it represents the most scientifically rigorous way to estimate directly the realistic impact of a community-based change in behaviour or some other modifiable exposure on the incidence of disease. This strength is enhanced when there are multiple intervention sites and multiple control sites. Weaknesses include a lack of rigid control over all the individuals in the trial, weaker standardization than RCT's in terms of entrance to the study, delivery of the intervention and monitoring of outcomes, and the small numbers of communities which are typically randomized, with consequent reductions in the chance of the treatment and control groups being comparable on both measured and unmeasured variables. In the long-term, geographical mobility (both into and out of the study communities) may lead to loss of effect and there is a danger that control communities in which nothing appears to be happening may become 'contaminated' by local campaigns to effect change.

Experiments of opportunity

In a **natural** or **quasi-experiment**, the researcher does not deliberately manipulate the supposed causal variable, but attempts to discover real-world situations in which the possibly causal variable has varied and then observes the effect of these changes on disease outcomes. This situation is often termed an **experiment of opportunity**. This design, despite the name, is an observational design, not a true experiment, as there is no possibility of randomization and the intervention is not planned with subsequent analysis in mind.

The most famous of all experiments of opportunity is John Snow's study of cholera. At the time of his research in the 1850s, there were two rival theories of cholera causation: the miasmic theory proposed that the cholera victim had breathed foul air which had been in contact with putrefied bodies and decaying vegetation. Snow believed that the disease was spread by drinking polluted water. He observed, in the 1849 outbreak, that cholera death rates were noticeably higher in those districts of London supplied by the Southwark–Vauxhall and Lambeth Water Companies. Both companies took their water from the Thames at a point that appeared to be polluted by sewage. Shortly before the 1854 epidemic, the Lambeth Company moved its intake to a less polluted reach at Thames Ditton. Clearly, if polluted water was the cause of cholera, one would expect those households supplied with this water to have a lower death rate. As Snow wrote:

> The experiment was on the grandest scale. No fewer than 300,000 people of both sexes, of every age and occupation, and of every rank and station, from gentlefolks down to the very poor were divided into two groups without their choice, and in most cases, without their knowledge; one group being supplied with water containing the sewage of London, the other group having water quite free from such impurity.
> (Snow [1855] 1936)

While the householders were often unable to tell Snow which company supplied their water, he was able to distinguish the suppliers on the basis of a chemical test. In a detailed examination of the first seven weeks of the 1854 epidemic, he showed that the mortality rate was over eight times higher in Southwark–Vauxhall-supplied houses than in the Lambeth-supplied houses (Table 4.2). Many years before, Robert Koch identified the cholera Vibrio in 1883, Snow was able to conclude that there was a 'cholera poison' that was transmitted by water.

While the innovative (and opportunistic and often just plain lucky) researcher can use natural experiments to subject relationships to an exacting test, it must be remembered they are not such powerful designs as randomized experiments. The population has not been allocated to

Table 4.2 Cholera deaths, first seven weeks of 1854 epidemic

Water-supply company	Number of houses	Cholera	Deaths per 10,000 houses
Southwark–Vauxhall	40,046	1263	315
Lambeth	26,107	98	37
Rest of London	256,423	1422	59

Source: data from Snow ([1855] 1936).

Table 4.3 CVD mortality, Monroe County, Florida, USA, 1940–50, rates per 100,000

	Rate	1940	1950	Percentage change
Monroe County	Crude	570	340	−40
	Age-adjusted	702	572	−18
	Age-sex-race-adjusted	684	575	−16
USA	Age-adjusted	508	440	−13

Source: data from Comstock 1979.

different groups prior to the changes in the exposure variable and, therefore, there may still be uncontrolled extraneous variables. A clear example of the dangers of overinterpretation is presented by the natural experiment on water-hardness and cardiovascular disease (CVD) mortality in Monroe County, Florida (Comstock 1979). In 1941, the Monroe County water supply was changed from very soft (0.5 parts per million) to hard (220 ppm) as deep well water was brought into use. If the hypothesis that hard water confers protection against CVD is correct, there should have been a decline in the CVD mortality rate given sufficient time. In fact, the rate appeared to drop dramatically, and within four years it was only a half of its 1941 level. But we must ask whether there were other confounding changes that accompanied the change to well water. Monroe County includes Key West Naval Base, and during and after the war there were major population changes in the area. As Table 4.3 shows, the crude CVD mortality rate did drop by nearly 50 per cent over ten years, but when account is taken of the changing composition of the population in terms of age, sex and race, the decline is much less. Initially impressive evidence for the water-hardness hypothesis is found to weaken when proper account is taken of confounding factors.

Conclusion

In this chapter we have reviewed the general principles which underpin epidemiologists' attempts to understand disease causation and examined what are widely held to be the most robust designs for achieving insight into the causes of disease. We have given particular consideration to the concept of causality, the notion of threats to validity, and the experimental design. A key to understanding the importance of the experimental design lies in the way in which it seeks closure and isolation. It focuses on one causal mechanism and one effect. It attempts closure so that only one mechanism is operating. Randomization and control are used to 'make all other things equal' and to isolate the one mechanism of interest. Such closure seldom occurs naturally as the real world is open to many different mechanisms operating at once.

Nevertheless, experimental design has an assured place in epidemiology and provides the basis for the current growth of evidence-based medicine in which evidence based on RCTs is generally accepted as being of the most trustworthy quality. While the ethical drawbacks of using RCTs with human subjects may be clear, there is also equally clear evidence of clinicians using treatments out of habit or for some other reason despite the RCTs having demonstrated that the clinicians are being ineffective – and in some ways unethical for disregarding sound scientific evidence. We return to this issue in Chapter 8; for the moment, however, it will suffice to note that the experimental design is scientifically sound but that its use in epidemiology is largely confined to the evaluation of new treatments for disease rather than hypotheses about disease causation.

Summary

- The chapter discusses the key principles underpinning analytical epidemiological designs.

- If a researcher wishes to draw causal inferences from a study, both exposure and disease should co-vary over space and time.

- Three general factors are recognized as reducing the internal validity of a study: bias (systematic error), confounding (another unrecognized variable influencing the observed results), and random error (chance). A study with low internal validity is worthless.

- Two basic types of randomized design are recognized: randomized clinical trials in which the basic unit of intervention is an individual subject, and community trials in which the basic unit of intervention is the group.

- Quasi-experimental designs often involve experiments of opportunity or natural experiments in which the exposure has changed naturally without the direct intervention of the researcher. Quasi-experimental designs are characterized by their lack of randomization.

Further reading

Bowling, A. (1997) *Research Methods in Health*. Buckingham: Open University Press, chapters 9 and 10.

Brownson, R. and Petitti, D. (eds) (1998) *Applied Epidemiology*. Oxford: Oxford University Press.

Jones, K. and Moon, G. (1987) *Health, Disease and Society*. London: Routledge, chapters 2 and 3.

Pocock, S. (1983) *Clinical Trials: A Practical Approach*. Chichester: John Wiley.

Activities

1 Epidemiology is replete with terminology. Throughout this part of the book you will encounter a large number of terms each with a distinctive meaning. You will find it extremely helpful to compile your own 'dictionary' of terms with a brief explanation as you proceed.

2 For a disease of your choice, draw an arrow diagram to show a multicausal relationship between exposures and outcome. Think how you would handle temporal precedence in determining cause and effect.

3 You have been asked to assist on a study in your professional area of occupational burnout (exhaustion leading to an inability to do a job effectively; it is generally accepted to be caused by lack of control over what takes place in the work environment).
   How would you:

   (a) select subjects to be included in the study;
   (b) measure disease status (burnout or not) in a consistent manner;
   (c) measure exposure status (control over work) in a consistent manner;
   (d) avoid recall bias?

   What problems would you anticipate in terms of:

   (e) interviewer bias;
   (f) unacceptability bias?

   What do you think are potentially important confounders? (To answer this question you will have to identify variables that are related to both the outcome and to the exposure.)

4 'Wonderdrug' has been invented. It is reputed to cure the major health problem that you encounter in your professional work. Can you think of a way to conduct an RCT to ascertain the effectiveness of 'Wonderdrug'? Try to devise a protocol for this experiment paying attention to sampling, the definition of control and intervention groups, randomization, blinding and ethics. Write your protocol as a series of steps and compare yours with that of a colleague working in the same area. Do you have areas of disagreement? If so, why?

5 What are the advantages and disadvantages of community trials when compared with individualized RCTs?

OBSERVATIONAL STUDIES AND DESIGN CHOICES

For some, the double-blind randomized trial is the only way to test a causal relationship with human subjects, and there is a tendency to disparage other designs. This is an unrealistic stance. Most of our understanding of human health in terms of treatment, cause and health care delivery comes from observational studies. Ethical considerations *generally* preclude an RCT when investigating disease causation. Consequently, we have to pay particular attention to how observational studies are designed and executed. We also need to be able to judge the appropriate design for a particular sort of research question.

By the end of this chapter, you should be able to:

- assess the relative strengths and weaknesses of observational designs in epidemiology;
- consider the practical difficulties inherent in implementing a particular design;
- choose an appropriate research design for a particular problem.

Before dealing with the specifics of the variety of different observational designs we will consider some general issues that apply to all such designs. In particular we will introduce a basic tabular device that allows us to make sense of different designs as well as providing a basis for the analytical techniques that are introduced in the next chapter. We must also acknowledge at the outset that the major weakness of observational designs is that there is no randomization. Consequently, all observational studies are open to the criticism that there are unknown confounders that have not been taken into account, and accordingly the results can be doubted.

Observational designs

It is common to distinguish between two main categories of observational design in epidemiology. *Descriptive designs* have already been introduced (Chapter 3). They provide information on patterns of disease, that is, on the frequency and distribution of disease in relation to other variables. They are crucial to the planning of health services, the allocation of resources, and to the monitoring of trends. They can also give clues to causes and determinants of disease, that is, they are hypothesis-generating. **Analytical designs** aim to identify associations between a disease and possible causes. They test hypotheses. There are three main types of analytical observational designs that can be distinguished by using what is known as a two-by-two table (Box 5.1).

Box 5.1 The basic 2 × 2 table for observational studies

		Exposure status		Total
		Yes	No	
Disease status	Yes	A	B	A + B
	No	C	D	C + D
	Total	A + C	B + D	N

It is worth taking a few minutes to become really familiar with this table, as it will recur in this and the next chapter in many guises. The columns in the table represent exposure status (yes or no), while the rows represent disease status (yes or no). The cells within the table, A, B, C and D, give the counts of the number of people with a particular combination of characteristics, so that A is the number of people who have been exposed and also have the disease. The row marginal totals, A+B and C+D, give the number of people who are diseased and healthy, respectively. The column marginal totals, A+C and B+D, give the number of people who are exposed and unexposed, respectively. The overall total, N, gives total number of subjects exposed and unexposed, diseased and healthy.

In terms of different analytical observational designs, **cohort studies** start by knowing the marginal totals of exposed (A+C) and non-exposed (B+D) subjects. These subjects are then monitored through time for the development of disease. The internal cells of the table are completed at the end of the follow-up period. **Case-comparison** or **case-control** studies begin with the column totals A+B (diseased cases) and C+D (healthy comparisons, or controls) and search for differences between the two groups in terms of past exposure to risk factors by completing the internal cell counts. *Cross-sectional studies*, which were encountered in Chapter 3 in a descriptive mode in the context of their use in determining prevalence, are sometimes used in hypothesis-testing mode. In such situations, information is collected on respondents for both current health status and exposure. This involves starting by selecting a sample (N), then ascertaining each subject's exposure and disease status, the internal cells, and finally calculating the marginal totals. As we have already considered cross-sectional studies in some depth, we will focus the remainder of this section on cohort and case comparison designs.

Cohort designs

A cohort design, like an experiment, is characterized by going from exposure to outcome, from cause to effect. Each selected subject is free from the disease when exposure status is defined and must be available for follow-up over a period of time, sometimes many years, in order to assess the occurrence of the disease. Cohort designs are observational studies because there is no allocation of exposure. They are analytical designs because they are usually confined to studies determining and investigating aetiological factors. Two subtypes are in common use and they are distinguished by how the samples are chosen:

- The one-sample cohort study starts with N subjects, the total of exposed (A+C) and non-exposed (B+D) subjects. This type of cohort study often involves the monitoring of a population over an extended period of time. It is useful for investigating multiple determinants and outcomes. A classic example is the Framingham Study in which residents of the town of Framingham in Massachusetts have been continuously monitored since 1950 with respect to many different risk factors and disease outcomes (Dawber *et al.* 1993). Another set of examples is provided by the British birth cohort studies. These involve every child born in a particular week in Britain in 1946, 1958 and 1970.
- The multisample cohort design involves selecting subgroups with known exposures, for example an exposed cohort (A+C) such those who have worked in a particular factory, and a non-exposed, comparison cohort (B+D). Such designs have been used to follow survivors of the atomic bomb explosions in Japan in 1945 and those affected by the Chernobyl nuclear plant accident in 1986.

Although the basic feature of all cohort studies is measurement of exposure and follow-up for disease, there are several variations depending on the *timing* of data collection. It is possible to distinguish three approaches as shown in Table 5.1. The purely **prospective design** is distinguished by determination of exposure levels at baseline (the present) and the subjects are followed for occurrence of disease at some time in the future. The **retrospective design** makes use of historical data to determine exposure level at some baseline in the past. The determination of disease status occurs in the present. This design is often used to research working environments and it obviously requires good historical records. The *historical prospective* or *ambispective design* uses both a retrospective view (to determine baseline exposure) and a prospective view (to determine disease incidence). To conduct such a study it must first be possible to identify

Table 5.1 Cohort designs and timing

Design	Past	Present	Future
Prospective	–	E	O
Retrospective	E	O	–
Ambispective	E	E	O

E = Exposure measurement; O = Outcome measurement

from records the membership of some previously existing group, such as all the employees of a given industry or all the students in a certain school at a specific date in the past. Secondly, it is necessary that the exposure of interest should have been recorded adequately at that time, or can be reconstructed from other sources. Thirdly, the cohort is then continued forward prospectively, adding new data as and when they happen to that assembled retrospectively.

Cohort studies in general have several clearly identified strengths. As participants are free of the disease at the outset, the time lag and temporal precedence between being exposed and diseased can be clearly established. They are moderately efficient for the study of rare exposures, particularly when the multisample approach is used, as it is possible to select cohorts with known exposures (such as certain occupational groups). Importantly, they also allow the examination of multiple effects from a single exposure, and can yield information on multiple exposures.

Purely prospective studies have additional advantages, as do retrospective cohorts. Prospective designs allow the researcher to access more recent information or acquire information directly from the subjects and have no problem of selection bias because exposure is assessed prior to the onset of the disease. Retrospective cohort designs are cheaper and quicker. Because the events have occurred before the study takes place, conclusions can be drawn more rapidly. They may also be the only feasible way to study the effects of exposures that no longer occur, such as those resulting from discontinued industrial processes.

These advantages are, however, matched by some major disadvantages. Cohort studies are very expensive and time consuming if large numbers of people are to be followed for many years. The required size of a cohort study depends not only on the size of the risk being investigated but also on the incidence of the particular condition under investigation. If a rare disease condition is investigated, very few events will be observed amongst many thousands of subjects whether exposed or not. The amount of time required to accumulate sufficient outcomes for meaningful analysis can be reduced by increasing the size of the cohort, but this increase has to be balanced against the longer time to assemble and measure the cohort as well as the increased financial and analytical costs. Thus attrition bias can increase with longer studies and have important impacts if those lost from the study are different in some way from those retained. Prospective cohort studies are particularly time consuming and expensive as there may be a very long wait before an exposure has any noticeable effect. They are very inefficient for the study of rare diseases, unless the study population is extremely large, and can also be prone to selection bias because knowledge of the disease outcome could influence the selection of exposed and unexposed individuals. Retrospective studies can be affected by selection bias as they rely on the availability of accurate information on both exposure and subsequent morbidity or mortality. There may also be problems due to the lack of records available on potential confounding factors and such studies are not useful for studying new types of exposure where past records will not exist.

All cohort designs require procedures to select the exposed and comparison groups, procedures to measure exposure and outcome, and protocols to ensure follow-up. For common exposures such as cigarette smoking, sufficient-sized samples of the exposed population can be found in the general population. An efficient design could follow prospectively only those in the extremes of the distribution of exposure, such as non-smokers and heavy smokers. Unusual exposures, such as the effects of a particular chemical, may indicate a need to work with more specific groups. It is common for exposure groups to be chosen for ease of selection both at the onset of the study and during follow-up. These include temporally defined groups, such as those born on specific days of the year, or all children born in a particular week of the year as in the birth cohort studies; geographically defined groups, such as the study of CHD in Framingham, Massachusetts; or certain occupational groups, such as general practitioners or military veterans where records are available and registration or pension schemes are maintained making long-term follow-up feasible.

The comparison group should be as similar to the exposed group as possible apart from their exposure to the causal factor under investigation. If several risk factors are under investigation simultaneously, it is important that the comparison group is unexposed on each of these factors. A majority of retrospective cohort studies use the general population as the unexposed comparison. This use of the general population for comparison can be misleading as a percentage of the general population may have been exposed. Moreover, in the case of occupational exposures, the general population tends to be less healthy than those in employment (the healthy worker effect). Consequently, the best advice is to select a comparison group from a demographically similar setting, but without the exposure.

When measuring exposure it is important that the information is gathered from comparable sources. It is also vital that potential confounding variables are measured as well as specific exposure variables. Provided they are recorded, differences in these baseline characteristics between groups can be allowed for during analysis. Similar strictures apply to the measurement of outcomes. Ensuring follow-up is perhaps the most important and difficult part of cohort study. Without comprehensive outcomes for both the exposed and control groups, the study is worthless. Unfortunately, this is very costly in terms of time, money and other resources.

As an example we briefly consider a retrospective cohort study of the effects of exposure to atmospheric nuclear weapons testing on serving troops (Pearce et al. 1990). Using records from the Royal New Zealand Navy, Pearce and co-workers defined an exposure group of 500 and a comparison group of navy personnel from three other ships who were on active service at the time (1957–58) but not involved in the testing. Data were obtained from death certificates, drivers' licence records, the national cancer registry, and a postal questionnaire which tried to find out if each respondent was dead, alive, or suffering from cancer. The study therefore represents a 30-year follow-up. It found a similar overall death rate in the two groups, but an excess of leukaemia in those exposed to the nuclear testing. The study has a problem, however, in that there is no real exposure information for the comparison sample. They could have been exposed to radiation exposure other than from these particular tests.

Case-comparison designs

Case-comparison designs are analytical observational studies in which subjects are selected on the basis of whether they have or do not have a particular disease. Typically a number of cases are identified and then some multiple of comparisons are subsequently identified. From the standpoint of selection of subjects, one is going from the effect to cause, from the outcome to the exposure. In terms of our standard tabulation, this study design aims to separate the row marginal totals (the cases and comparisons) into the internal cells which signify the joint disease and exposure status (Box 5.2). The box deliberately does not show the column marginal totals A+C and B+D, or the total N, for these totals are meaningless. The study selects only some subset of the total population, namely the cases and some number of controls. Another distinctive feature of the design is that there is only one observation point: cases and controls are selected, and data are collected about past exposures that may have contributed to disease.

Box 5.2 The case-comparison design

| | | Exposure status | | Total |
		Yes	No	
Disease status	Yes	A	B	A + B
	No	C	D	C + D

Perhaps the most striking example of an effective case-control study is that which identified thalidomide used during pregnancy as causing limb malformations in babies. Mellin and Katzenstein (1962) identified 46 cases of malformed babies born in Germany during 1959 and 1960. Their mothers' thalidomide exposure was compared with that of 300 mothers of normal babies, finding that 41 of the cases had been exposed to the drug compared with none of the controls.

Traditionally, case-comparison and cohort studies have been portrayed as very different designs, with the former being a generally inferior alternative. However, inherent in the case-comparison is the notion of a more-or-less explicit follow-up study within which the case-comparison is nested.

Indeed, the only conceptual distinction between a cohort and a case-comparison is that of studying the entire cohort's experience over time versus sampling from this experience. The objective in designing the case-comparison is therefore to obtain the same result as the corresponding follow-up study would have given. Consequently, the case-comparison approach will not compromise the validity of results unless there has been a biased selection of cases or comparisons. Case-comparison designs are simply studies in which there is a different sampling fraction for cases and comparisons. The proportion of persons in the study who have the disease is no longer determined by the disease risk in the source population, but rather by the choice of the investigator. That is, a disease that occurs infrequently in the source population can be over-sampled, so that affected individuals constitute a large proportion of the study sample. This ability to over-sample affected individuals is why case-control studies are statistically efficient for the study of rare diseases.

There are two commonly used variants on the case-comparison design. In the **matched design** the comparisons are chosen to match individual cases for certain important variables such as age and sex. In the *unmatched design* the comparisons are selected without any attention to matching. In both situations there can be just one comparison for each case, but if cases are difficult to collect while comparisons are relatively plentiful, some multiple can be used. However, it is known that there is little gain in efficiency by selecting more than five times as many comparisons as cases.

Matching is a much more complex technique than it appears, as it can be used (and misused) to achieve three different purposes:

- to increase efficiency and reduce sample size
- to limit confounding
- to improve the comparability of collected information.

Any characteristic of an individual, such as age, sex, neighbourhood, class, occupation, personal or family history of disease may serve as a basis for matching. In individual matching, each individual in the case group is paired with a similar individual in the comparison group. For example, we could have a male 25-year-old civil servant in both groups thereby matching on age, sex and occupation. This is often difficult to achieve exactly and 'frequency' matching can then be used. Thus if there are ten white-collar males aged between 30 and 40 in the cases group, there would need to be a similar frequency in the comparison group. This approach is also used when matching is done on a continuous variable such as blood pressure: a blood-pressure range is used to achieve frequency matching.

Normally it is recommended that matching is limited to no more than three variables which are known to influence outcome, common variables being age, sex and social class. Such matching allows for the control of potentially confounding variables and allows smaller sample sizes to be used. In a case-comparison study, individual matching in the design must be followed through in the analysis. Any variable that is matched cannot be analysed for its effect on a disease outcome, as the matching will mean that any effect will be removed by design. The cases will, by definition, be similar to the comparisons on the matched variables. Matching is thus inappropriate for an exploratory study in which it is wished to answer a general question as to what are the causes of the outcome in question.

The practicalities of the case-comparison design involve selecting cases and comparisons, and measuring disease and exposure status. The initial problems are to define a case conceptually, and to identify a case operationally. At issue is misclassification. The researcher's aim is to ensure that all genuine cases have an equal probability of entering the study and that no false case is included. The literature suggests that benefits of a more restrictive definition of a case outweigh the benefits of being overly inclusive. This indicates a need to work on as homogeneous a disease entity as possible and to establish strict diagnostic criteria for the disease.

The ideal situation is to work with incidence cases (see Chapter 1) in a defined population in a specified time period. With prevalence cases it can become difficult to separate the cause of the disease from those factors that affect duration and survivorship. Moreover, with incident cases there is likely to be better recall of past exposures and a reduced chance that exposure has changed as a consequence of the disease. Temporal sequence between exposure and disease is always an issue in case-control studies, and this becomes an even more serious problem when prevalent cases are used. Since diagnostic fashions change over time, recent diagnoses should be more uniform than those drawn from different time periods. In contrast, the advantage of prevalence cases is that it is often easy to increase the sample size available for study. This may be particularly important for rare diseases. Overall, a balance is required: inclusion criteria are chosen to minimize misclassification yet allow for a feasible study.

In practice, cases are usually selected from two sources: hospitals and the general community. A hospital-based case-comparison study uses patients who have received treatment during a specific period of time. This can be relatively easy and inexpensive to put into action. In contrast, in a population-based study, potential cases are all persons with disease in a defined population at a single point or during a given period of time. This can be expensive and time consuming (particularly if the disease is rare), as it involves locating and obtaining data from all affected individuals or a random, cross-sectional sample from the defined population. Community cases, however, have two advantages over hospital-derived cases. First, they avoid bias arising from whatever selection factors lead an affected individual to go to a particular doctor or hospital/surgery. Secondly, they allow description of the entire picture of disease in that population and direct computation of rates.

The choice of an appropriate comparison is perhaps the most critical issue in designing a case-comparison study. Comparisons are needed to evaluate whether the frequency of an exposure or specified characteristic observed in the case group is different from that which would be expected based on experience of a series of comparable individuals who do not have the disease. It is worthwhile considering what is the *ideal* comparison. To avoid confounding, such a comparison would have the same characteristics as the cases, with the single exception of the exposure of interest. The most clear-cut evidence that an exposure is indeed causal is when the cases and comparisons are all the same age and sex, eat the same food, work in the same environment and so on, but all of the cases are exposed and none of the comparisons are exposed. Cases and controls should have the same *opportunity* for exposure. Thus, if the cases were all treated in one particular hospital, the controls should represent people who, had they developed the disease, would also have gone to the same hospital. If you want to generalize from the study to the general population, it is important that comparisons are representative of the general population in terms of probability of exposure to the risk factor.

Practice is often far from this ideal and compromised by practicalities and logistics. Three distinct approaches can be identified:

- *Hospital comparisons*: these are patients who are being treated for conditions other than the disease being studied. The advantages of hospital comparisons are that they are easily identifiable and readily available in sufficient numbers. Because they are receiving treatment, they are also more likely than the general population to be aware of previous exposures and events, thereby decreasing the potential for recall bias. They are more likely to have experienced the same intangible selection factors that influenced cases to seek medical care and they are also, because they are receiving treatment, more likely to be willing to cooperate, thereby reducing non-response bias. Their disadvantages are that they may not be representative of the true exposure rates in the target population. Hospital comparisons are people who are ill enough to seek medical attention and can therefore be expected to differ from the general population in terms of other confounding risk factors such as smoking or being overweight. Although hospitalized patients may generally share the same selective processes by which cases are identified, this is not equally true for all diseases, and this leads to the main difficulty of using hospital controls, which is trying to decide the diagnostic categories from which to select the comparisons. In general, hospital-based comparisons are inherently subject to greater potential for error than population-based studies but their use is justified when little information has been reported about a particular exposure–disease association and when a population-based case registry is not available.
- *Special comparisons*: friends, relatives and neighbours of the cases are sometimes used as comparisons. The advantage of these 'special' groups is that they generally share the advantages of general population comparisons, while being much easier to contact and recruit. They can also offer a degree of control for confounding factors such as ethnic background, social class and environment. However, they can give an underestimate of the true effect of exposure if the study factor is one for which family members and friends are likely to be too similar to the cases (that is *overmatched*). Indeed, one may end up controlling for an important (unidentified) risk factor that could no longer be evaluated.
- *Population comparisons*: comparisons from the general population are normally obtained by the usual methods of random sampling rather than matching. If used with community-based cases they have a very high degree of comparability. Random selection should result in a comparison group that is representative of the exposure rate in the general population. In practice, however, there may be major logistical difficulties in that population comparisons are costly and time consuming and the

quality of information may differ between cases and comparisons. Healthy individuals may be less motivated to participate as comparisons, resulting in the need to contact more individuals and a study which rapidly becomes more expensive. Finally, the use of population comparisons may confer selection bias in that those who refuse or cannot be contacted may systematically differ from participants in a way related to the risk of developing the disease.

Each source of comparison has its own merits and limitations. It is sometimes desirable to form two or more distinct control series from different sources and to compare results among them. If one has a procedure for ascertaining all incident cases occurring within a geographical area in a defined period of time, then the use of comparisons selected at random from the general population is undoubtedly the option of choice. With a properly designed and implemented sampling procedure, an unbiased selection of comparisons can be assured. Furthermore, the absolute risks of disease associated with the presence or absence of exposure can often be determined, because the size of the populations at risk is frequently known from the census or other information.

Disease and exposure status can be obtained through workplace or medical records, interviews and examinations. The interviews can be with subjects themselves, or through a surrogate such as their partner or employer. Owing to the problems of bias, it is wise to try to blind interviewers to case/comparison status of subjects, ensure that they are unaware of specific hypotheses being tested, and use standardized procedures. Interviews can deal with a wide range of potential risk factors while the costs are relatively low. In order to minimize problems associated with subject recall, you can attempt to corroborate exposures through other methods, such as an interview as well as records. The amount of information found in records is often limited, however, and the quality variable.

Case-comparison studies are quick and inexpensive compared with other analytical designs. This is because they tend to be smaller in size, and they often use existing data. As a result of this efficiency, case-comparisons are likely to be replicated. They are particularly well suited to the evaluation of diseases with long latent periods as the start point is a group of people who have the disease; there is no question of waiting for the disease to develop or manifest itself. They are also optimal for research on rare diseases, as subjects are selected on disease status, thereby allowing investigators to identify adequate numbers of diseased and non-diseased individuals. For example, suppose you wish to investigate the association between a rare birth defect and mothers' smoking. If the proportion of outcomes is 1 per cent and 25 per cent of the mothers smoke there would need to be 5000 mothers in a cohort study to get 50 cases. It may be shown that a case-comparison study of 100 cases and 100 controls will give approximately the same efficiency (McNeil 1996). The design is especially useful in the early stage of development of knowledge about a disease when trying to untangle competing and interacting ideas about disease causation.

On the negative side, case-comparisons can be very inefficient for the evaluation of rare *exposures*. Despite a large number of cases, one may still end up with few exposed cases, unless the exposure is common amongst those with the disease. In moving from the effect (disease) to cause (previous exposure), the temporal relationship between exposure and disease may also be difficult to establish. Compared with cohort studies, case-comparison epidemiology is particularly prone to systematic error, especially selection and recall bias. Consequently, there is a need to guard against differential selection of cases and comparisons and differential reporting or recording of exposure information. Cases suffering a disease are likely to be more motivated to recall possible risk factors, and this recall bias has often been a major source of criticism.

As case-comparison studies are relatively quick and easy to do for multiple exposures and risks, there is a temptation to adopt a 'shotgun' approach: to try a large number of different hypotheses to see if anything comes up. However, the larger the number of hypotheses that are evaluated simultaneously the greater the chance of finding something just by chance. This approach is also known as data-dredging, fishing, or slightly more politely as data-derived hypotheses. While this approach is tempting and can be useful when little is known about the disease, there is also a subsequent need for more rigorous evaluation on an independent dataset with a study designed to address that specific question. The real problem comes when you actually carry out a shotgun approach but report only the positive findings.

Choosing between designs

Cohort, case-comparison and cross-sectional designs are fundamentally distinguished only by the method of selection of subjects. In a cross-sectional study, subjects are selected from a population without regard to exposure or outcome. In a cohort study, the subjects are selected before they experience the outcome, and different selection criteria may be used for different exposure categories in the multisample variant of this design. In a case-comparison design, cases are chosen that have experienced the outcome, as well as comparisons that have not; differential selection criteria may be used for the cases and the controls. Box 5.3 gives the variety of names that are used for these different designs and their basic variants in the epidemiological literature. The rest of this chapter consolidates information on each design and considers their relative advantages and disadvantages. This approach is intended to help you to appreciate the issues that need attention when choosing among designs.

No one type of study design is uniformly superior to the others in every situation, and any appropriate choice depends on several factors including the rarity of the disease, its latency and duration and how much is already known of the aetiology of the disease. Each of the designs has drawbacks and advantages and these are listed for the three most commonly used designs in Table 5.2. Before making some recommendations, we shall return to some of the threats of validity which we discussed in the previous chapter, and consider four issues: temporal relations, recall bias, rarity and cost.

Box 5.3   Some equivalences in the 'terminology jungle'

Interventionist study   = Randomized trial   = Experimental study
Randomized clinical trial   = RCT
Community trial   = Group trial   = Community intervention trial
Experiments of opportunity   = Quasi-experiment   = Natural experiment

Cohort design   = Follow-up study   = Longitudinal study
Purely prospective design   = Concurrent cohort study = Prospective cohort design
Retrospective cohort   = Historical cohort study = Non-current cohort
Historical prospective cohort = Ambispective

Case-comparison study   = Case-control   = Retrospective study

Cross-sectional study   = Geographical study   = Prevalence survey

---

Table 5.2   Advantages (A) and disadvantages (D) of three observational designs

	Cross-sectional	Case-comparison	Prospective cohort
Many hypotheses to test		A	D
Rare diseases	D	A	D
Selective recall of important events		D	A
Attrition (death, migration, loss of participation)	A	A	D
Non-response	D	A	D
Time needed to complete study	A	A	D
Cost		A	D
Inference to population	A	D	A
Temporal relation of aetiological factor and disease onset	D	D	A
Establishing directness of association	D	D	A
Selection of controls leading to bias		D	A

Source: after Roht 1982: 384.

An important element in the choice of a design is the temporal relationship between the possible causal factors and the disease. When the causal factor and disease are measured simultaneously, it is impossible to discover whether the possible cause actually preceded the occurrence of the disease. For example, if it is found in a cross-sectional study that people who have suffered a stroke have a high cholesterol level, the researcher cannot ascertain whether this high value preceded or followed the stroke. Case-comparisons and cohort studies are much stronger in this area.

Cross-sectional, case-comparisons and cohorts involving retrospective elements may involve memory distortion or recall bias; the presence of disease may heighten or lower the recall of certain events. For example, the patient with cirrhosis of the liver may underestimate the amount of alcohol consumed over the past 30 years. In a prospective cohort study, the information collected cannot be biased by the outcome of diseases for it has not yet happened, but, conversely, data collection may inadvertently influence behaviour.

With rare diseases, cross-sectional and cohort designs are difficult to perform and a very large sample followed over a long period may be needed to uncover just a few cases. For example, the Royal College of General Practitioners has estimated that it would require some 125,000 person-years of use to identify significantly different rates of pulmonary embolism in oral contraceptive users and non-users. Similarly, it has been estimated that 100,000 individuals would be needed in a cohort study with a prevalence of 1 per 1000 for the unexposed group and 2 per 1000 for the exposed. For very rare conditions, the only feasible type of study is the case-comparison.

This issue of data efficiency is closely related to the cost and speed of the study: case-comparisons are usually the quickest and cheapest to do, while prospective cohort studies are the most expensive and are subject to long delays.

Conclusion

In the light of these comments and the information of Table 5.2, it is possible to make some general recommendations. The cross-sectional approach is best suited to discovering the extent of a problem and exploratory work when little is known about the aetiology of a disease. It is ideal for determining the burden of disease. Such studies form a valuable and essential supplement to routine data, and they need not necessarily be time consuming or expensive.

Case-comparison studies are useful for the rapid testing of a **hypothesis**, particularly for rare diseases, but care must be taken to guard against recall and selection bias. They permit the testing of several hypotheses at once and provide preliminary support for tentative explanations. On the whole, cohort studies have tended to confirm associations uncovered by the case-comparisons methods.

The cohort study is not good at generating ideas and is unsuitable for rare diseases, but the multisample form is excellent for rare exposures. Providing there is no participation or attrition bias, this design allows rigorous testing of causal hypotheses derived from other studies. It is most useful when specific hypotheses are well developed and supported by previous studies and final, additional evidence is required.

When relatively little is known, study designs that use existing data, that are quick and easy to conduct, and are economical are to be preferred. However, as understanding increases, and the complexity and specificity of the research questions increase, then more rigorous study designs are required. We can recognize *epidemiological study cycles* in which an initial pattern is found in either a few clinical cases or through an analysis of routine data. Initial hypotheses are evaluated in case-comparison studies, or retrospective cohort studies. If support is found and risk factors identified,

THE DESIGN AND ANALYSIS OF EPIDEMIOLOGICAL STUDIES

of a birth or death. In both cases, a data collection form is needed and the principles governing the design of these forms are fairly universal.

There are numerous texts on survey methods and it is not our purpose here to provide an exhaustive guide to how to do surveys. Interested readers should consult a classic specialist textbook such as Moser and Kalton (1971) or Hoinville *et al.* (1977). The key points to bear in mind, either when conducting your own survey, or when evaluating someone else's – or even when thinking about the ways in which **routine statistics** are originated – are:

- *Concept clarity*: are concepts explained clearly at the data collection stage and is there a shared understanding of what they mean? This might involve the wording of questions and the development of protocols to ensure that there are clear definitions of concepts.
- *Sampling*: while routine data should clearly cover users of services and those events where registration is required, other sources, with the exception of the national census of the population, will necessitate the sampling of some fraction of the population. This approach reflects practicality as well as a recognition that you seldom need to ask something of everyone before you have a good idea what the pattern of responses will be. The sampling method of choice is **random sampling**. With this method, individuals have an equal probability of being chosen and are selected from a larger sampling frame using

---

Box 2.1 A note on categorical and continuous data

Categorical data refer to counts in categories or classes. They are usually presented in tabular form such as:

	Exposed to known carcinogen	Not exposed to known carcinogen
Cancer present	7	5
Cancer not present	27	29

Each value in each *cell* of the table represents a count of people who have the characteristic defined by that cell's row and column. In the above, the count of 27, for example, represents 27 people who do not have cancer but have been exposed to a known carcinogen. Such data are often also termed *nominal* data.

Continuous data provide an exact position on a continuous scale and are not represented as counts in categories. Examples include a person's height (m) or weight (kg), the number of deaths from a certain cause per year in a region (deaths per year), toxic emissions from a factory chimney (tonnes per year) or the amount spent by a company on health and safety training (£ per year). A researcher has much more analytical scope with continuous data but may decide to convert it to nominal to aid in its description or summary.

EPIDEMIOLOGICAL INFORMATION

Data are the very life-blood of epidemiology. Epidemiologists can use data that have been collected and published by others (**secondary data**) or collect their own data by conducting surveys, for example (**primary data**). There is a wide range of survey techniques and research designs that can be used to collect data. The research designs are described in Part 2 of the book. In this chapter we present a brief review of survey method but aim primarily to provide a review of sources of routine secondary health-related data. We also present an assessment of the value and limitations of routine sources and give some consideration to the secondary use of social surveys that collect health-related data.

At the end of the chapter you should:

- have an appreciation of the range of routine secondary data available for epidemiological research;
- understand the limitations and drawbacks of such data.

Collecting epidemiological data

The research designs which we go on to consider in the rest of Part 1 provide the basic frameworks for the collection of epidemiological data. In a mechanical and operational sense, however, the collection of epidemiological data depends on survey methods. Here we use the term 'survey' very broadly to contain not only questionnaires completed by an individual, either in their right or by someone acting on their behalf, but also the many instruments which have been devised for the collection of routine information about health-related events such as the use of a hospital or the registration a prospective intervention trial may be designed to assess whether modification of such factors is possible and whether this is followed by reduction in disease. Table 5.3 brings all these considerations together and provides a summary of the strengths and weaknesses of the epidemiological study designs covered in this and the preceding chapter. Having set out the principles of these study designs, our attention now shifts to a consideration of the basic techniques for analysing the resulting epidemiological data.

Summary

- The basic feature of all cohort studies is the measurement of exposure and follow-up for disease outcome. There are several variations depending on the timing of data collection.

- Case-comparison designs are studies in which subjects are selected on the basis of whether they have or do not have a particular disease. A distinctive feature of the design is that there is only one observation point: cases and controls are selected, and data are collected about past exposures that may have contributed to disease.

- Cohort, case-comparison and cross-sectional designs are fundamentally distinguished only by the method of selection of subjects. However, they each have clear strengths and weaknesses.

Further reading

As with the two preceding chapters, follow-up reading is best undertaken by selective study of relevant chapters in other introductions to epidemiology, for example:

Brownson, R. and Petitti, D. (eds) (1998) *Applied Epidemiology.* Oxford: Oxford University Press.
Hennekens, C. and Buring, J. (1987) *Epidemiology in Medicine.* Boston: Little Brown.
Rothman, K. (1986*) Modern Epidemiology.* Boston: Little Brown.
Unwin, N., Carr, S. and Leeson, J. with Pless-Mulloli, T. (1997) *An Introductory Study Guide to Public Health and Epidemiology.* Buckingham: Open University Press.

Activities

1 You are interested in the hypothesis that the consumption of red wine can protect one from heart disease. Try to write a protocol to study this hypothesis using a cohort design. You will need to think about which sort of cohort design to use and the timing of the study as well as the

Table 5.3 Main properties of different designs

Design	Intervention trials	Cohort studies	Case-comparisons	Cross-sectional surveys
• Question asked	What is the effect of this intervention?	What are the effects of this exposure?	What were the causes of this event?	How common is this condition? Are conditions and exposures associated?
• Applicability	Controlled interventions of likely benefit	Any exposure for which adequate numbers of exposed subjects can be found and studies, and for which outcome can be assessed	Any event for which groups of cases and appropriate controls can be found, and for which exposure factors can be assessed retrospectively	Any exposure, condition or association which is reasonably common and for which assessment at one point in time is sufficient
• Major strengths	Primary method of studying new therapies	Primary method of studying unusual or new exposures	Primary method of studying unusual or new outcomes	Primary method of assessing prevalence
	Allows randomization – best way to control confounding Allows double-blind assessment – best way to control bias	Allows multiple endpoints to be assessed Cause to effect time sequence clear All measures of risk can be assessed Exposure is assessed prior to outcome, avoiding bias	Can usually be done with moderate numbers of subjects; feasible even on small numbers Retrospective method is rapid Multiple exposure factors can be assessed	Representative samples of a population can be drawn Methods can be standardized, reliable and single-blind Efficient in resources needed Cooperation may be high Can be repeated using similar methods
• Major weaknesses	Ethical limitations Organizational problems Timescale	Usually requires large numbers Long timescale for some effects	Retrospective method limits exposure information, and is open to bias Adequate control group may be difficult to define or obtain	Lack of time dimension limits causal interpretations Inefficient for rare exposures or conditions

Source: Elwood 1998.

definition of exposure and the measurement of outcome. Your protocol will need to justify your decisions on each of these issues and draw attention to any potential problems.

2 Repeat activity 1 but this time devise a case-comparison design. How would you define your cases (incidence or prevalance)? How would you select your comparisons? What would be important matching factors?

3 On balance, which design would you recommend? If you want, you could temporarily skip to Chapter 8 and read about literature searching. You could then use your local NHS or university library to search out studies on red wine and heart disease to see what designs they have used.

THE EPIDEMIOLOGICAL ANALYSIS OF TABULAR DATA

This chapter is concerned with the processing and analysis of epidemiological data and focuses on converting raw research *data* into more meaningful epidemiological *information*. Doing a study according to one of the designs outlined in the three preceding chapters is only part of the task. Sense has to be made of the data that have been collected.

Chapters 2 and 3 have already introduced some of the more fundamental statistical and graphical techniques used in the description, summary and analysis of what we have called *continuous* epidemiological data. Here attention focuses on the analysis of tabular data such as are collected from studies employing the standard epidemiological tabulation used in the previous two chapters. We will introduce a number of analytical techniques but particular attention is given to the calculation of *risk* and *odds*, two measures that are widely used in epidemiological analyses. We will also describe how confidence intervals can be generated for such measures. A section then describes methods for testing for *confounding* variables.

By the end of the chapter you should be able to:

- understand the underlying concepts behind epidemiological analyses;
- interpret results from epidemiological studies;
- critically evaluate published work;
- undertake a simple epidemiological analysis.

While continuous data are important in epidemiological studies, it is more common to focus on presence/absence data in terms of the relationship between exposure and outcome. Here attention is given to the analysis of data from *analytical* designs that aim to identify associations between diseases and possible causes. The 2 × 2 table of disease status versus exposure can represent all such designs. In these studies, the interest usually focuses on comparisons, that is knowing how the incidence in the exposed group, such as smokers, compares with the incidence in the non-exposed, the non-smokers.

Risk and odds

One of the key concepts in the quantitative approach discussed here is risk (and hence prevention of risk) and the related concept of the odds. Three main types of risk can be defined: absolute, relative and attributable.

Absolute risk and odds

Absolute risk is the risk for the whole population under study and equates with incidence proportion (see Chapter 3). If the risk of dying from a particular disease is known to be 0.3 (a three in ten chance), the risk or probability of survival is 1 − 0.3 = 0.7. Often in epidemiology it is common to use not just the risk in studying incidence, but a closely related concept that is defined in terms of the **odds**. Odds are a ratio of the probability of dying (or becoming ill) to the probability of surviving (or remaining well). Table 6.1 summarizes how these concepts interrelate.

In cohort studies both the odds and absolute risk are calculable directly, and it is easy to move between them. Indeed, when epidemiology is concerned with rare events in a given time period, that is events with a small risk of probability, both values are numerically very similar. With rare events, 1 minus the risk must be very close to 1, and the odds and the

Table 6.1 Absolute risk, probability of survival, and odds

Absolute risk	Probability of survival	Odds
0.90	1 − 0.90	$\dfrac{0.90}{1-0.9} = 9.0$
0.75	1 − 0.75	$\dfrac{0.75}{1-0.75} = 3.0$
0.50	1 − 0.50	$\dfrac{0.50}{1-0.50} = 1.0$
0.25	1 − 0.25	$\dfrac{0.25}{1-0.25} = 0.33$
0.10	1 − 0.10	$\dfrac{0.10}{1-0.10} = 0.11$
0.01	1 − 0.01	$\dfrac{0.01}{1-0.01} = 0.01$

risk parameters are nearly equal. This concept is often called the 'rare *disease* assumption' but this is really a misnomer because it should refer to the event not the disease *per se*. Even the most common and prevalent of diseases such as the common cold can be treated as a rare event if the time interval is short. When this is the case, the approximation is a reasonable one: when the risk is 0.01, the risk and the odds are approximately the same.

Relative risk

An epidemiologist is usually interested in differential risks for different exposures; not absolute risk but **relative risk**. In essence, the relative risk is used to compare the incidence of a disease or condition in a group possessing a particular attribute or exposure to those without. These types of comparisons can be made with case-comparison studies or cohort studies. The relative risk (RR) indicates the magnitude of the increased risk derived from the exposure. It does not relate to the absolute risk (AR) because situations can arise where the RR is high and the AR is low. Two forms of relative risk can be defined:

● *Risk ratio*: preferred term if prevalence or cumulative incidence proportions are compared.
● *Rate ratio*: preferred term if incidence density rates are compared.

Relative risk: the risk ratio

The risk ratio for the standard 2×2 table can be calculated directly and simply as the ratio of the risks (or incidence proportions) for the exposed to the non-exposed group. Box 6.1 sets out the necessary calculations.

Box 6.1   Risk ratio calculation

		Exposure status		Total
		Yes	No	
Disease	Yes	A	B	A + B
status	No	C	D	C + D
	Total	A + C	B + D	N

Incidence proportion in exposed = A/(A+C)
Incidence proportion in unexposed = B/(B+D)

$$\text{Risk ratio} = \frac{\text{Incidence proportion in exposed}}{\text{Incidence proportion in unexposed}}$$

$$RR = \frac{A/(A+C)}{B/(B+D)}$$

We can recognize three distinct interpretations of our result:

- If the RR is equal to 1, there is no association; there is no difference in the incidence proportion for the exposed and the unexposed.
- If the RR is greater than 1, there is a greater risk in the exposed group which may be causal, that is a positive association.
- If the RR is less than 1, there is a negative association so that exposure may possibly be protective.

Typically the risk ratios observed in empirical work have a small range. In environmental epidemiology, a relative risk greater than 2 or 3 is considered high. A relative risk of 2 indicates that the incidence rate of disease is two times higher in the exposed group than in the unexposed. Equivalently, this represents a 100 per cent increase in risk. A relative risk of 0.25 indicates a 75 per cent reduction in the incidence rate in exposed individuals as compared with the unexposed.

Box 6.2 shows the results obtained from a follow-up of the Health and Lifestyle Survey which relates to middle-aged men. The table shows the exposure status for 1224 (N) male subjects aged 41 to 60 in 1984, and their outcome status, dead or not, 13 years later in 1997. The incidence proportion for the smokers is 0.20, that is 20 per cent of the smokers have died; while the incidence proportion for the non-smokers is 0.12; only 12 per cent have died. The resultant relative risk for smokers to non-smokers is 1.65, showing an elevated risk for smokers – a 65 per cent increase in risk.

Box 6.2 Risk ratio for middle-aged men: smokers versus non-smokers (original analysis based on HALS data)

		Smoker 1984		
		Yes	No	Total
Dead 1997	Yes	88	92	180
	No	362	682	1044
	Total	450	774	1224

$$RR = \frac{88/(88+362)}{92/(92+682)} = \frac{0.195}{0.118} = 1.65$$

Relative risk: the rate ratio

Whereas the risk ratio involves the comparison of incidence proportions, the rate ratio compares incidence-density rates. Thus the rate ratio compares the rate of development of new cases per person-time in the exposed population with the rate of development in the unexposed population. The interpretation remains the same, so that a rate ratio of greater than 1 suggests an increased relative risk for the exposed group. Box 6.3 shows the data derived from a 20-year follow-up of British general practitioners in terms of the initial exposure: smoker and non-smoker (Doll and Peto 1976).

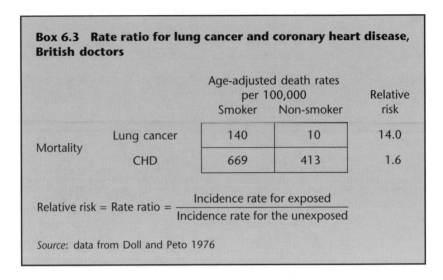

Box 6.3   Rate ratio for lung cancer and coronary heart disease, British doctors

		Age-adjusted death rates per 100,000		Relative risk
		Smoker	Non-smoker	
Mortality	Lung cancer	140	10	14.0
	CHD	669	413	1.6

$$\text{Relative risk} = \text{Rate ratio} = \frac{\text{Incidence rate for exposed}}{\text{Incidence rate for the unexposed}}$$

Source: data from Doll and Peto 1976

The risk ratio for lung cancer is derived as the incidence density of the smokers to non-smokers, that is 140 per 100,000 divided by 10 per 100,000 giving a risk ratio of 14.0. The equivalent figure for coronary heart disease is 1.6. The value of 14.0 is a very high one indeed; even the ratio of 1.6 suggests a substantially increased risk. This particular rate ratio is probably the most reported result in epidemiology.

Relative risk and the odds ratio

In the same way that odds can be calculated alongside absolute risk, an *odds ratio* (OR) can also be calculated for the 2×2 table to assess differential exposure in cohort designs. The basic 2×2 table is again shown in Box 6.4 with the formula for the odds ratio, (sometimes known as *relative odds*) included. The odds of the diseased or dying group being exposed is A/B, while the odds for the well or surviving group being exposed are C/D. The odds ratio is interpreted in a similar manner to the relative risk, where:

- a value of 1 indicates that there are no increased or decreased odds associated with the disease;
- a value greater than 1 suggests that those with the disease (or those who die) have an increased odds of exposure;
- a value less than 1 suggests that the exposure could be protective.

The calculations using the actual data shown in Box 6.2 are presented on the bottom line of Box 6.4. The relative odds of being a smoker for those who die compared with those who survive is 1.802. Those men who died had higher odds of being a smoker (that is, are more likely to have been smokers) than those who survived.

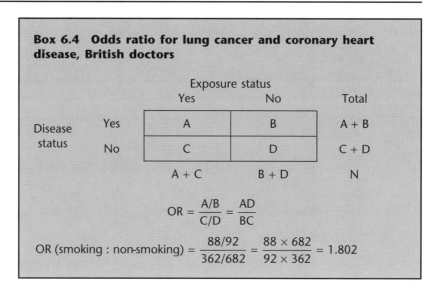

Box 6.4 Odds ratio for lung cancer and coronary heart disease, British doctors

| | | Exposure status | | |
		Yes	No	Total
Disease status	Yes	A	B	A + B
	No	C	D	C + D
		A + C	B + D	N

$$OR = \frac{A/B}{C/D} = \frac{AD}{BC}$$

$$OR \text{ (smoking : non-smoking)} = \frac{88/92}{362/682} = \frac{88 \times 682}{92 \times 362} = 1.802$$

In a cohort study, both the relative odds and the relative risk are appropriate measures although there is a tendency to report the RR in preference to the OR. When the study is dealing with rare events, the relative risk and the odds ratio will be approximately the same.

Relative risk: extensions and limits

In terms of exposure, a binary outcome has been used so far, such as smoker or not. This, however, could easily have been refined into several categories. For example, the categories: none, light (1–5), medium (6–20) and heavy (21+) could have been used to categorize the amount smoked. One of the levels of exposure is then taken as a base and the other categories are compared with this base to derive relative risks and odds. It is usual to choose the group with what is thought to be the lowest risk (in this case the non-smoker category) to act as the base for comparison. The RR and OR of dying for each level of exposure could then be calculated by comparing data for each level of exposure with the unexposed category. Attention then focuses only on relative risks or odds ratios in excess of 1. This provides a powerful means of extending the utility of the RR and OR approach.

Conceptually a different problem but with an equivalent technical solution is when there is more than one exposure. Consider middle-aged men with two binary exposures: smoking versus non-smoking, and poor versus healthy diet. The base category is taken as a subject who eats healthily and does not smoke. The other three categories are contrasted against this base. The relative risk is calculated as shown in Box 6.5 by dividing the incidence rate for each of the three categories by the incidence rate for the base. The summary data suggest that the worst relative risk is when poor diet is combined with smoking. A poor diet on its own does not lead to a much increased risk. This is a case of a fourfold (2 × 2) classification of exposure, and theoretically the approach could be extended to more and more types and levels of exposure, so that we could examine the relative risk for four categories of smoking, two levels of diet and three levels of alcohol consumption in a model that requires 4 × 2 × 3 (= 24) terms to be estimated. If all these terms are to be reliably estimated a very large dataset is required.

Box 6.5   Analysis of multiple relative risks

Exposure category

Smoking	Poor Diet	Dead	Alive	Total	Risk	RR
No	No	57	427	484	0.12	1.00
Yes	No	38	166	204	0.19	1.58
No	Yes	35	255	290	0.12	1.00
Yes	Yes	50	196	246	0.20	1.67

$$RR = \frac{\text{Incidence for exposure category}}{\text{Incidence for base category}}$$

e.g. RR for smoker with poor diet $= \dfrac{0.20}{0.12} = 1.67$

On a more cautionary note, the astute reader will have recognized that our discussion of RR has been couched exclusively in terms of the cohort study design. It has been shown how the relative risk can be calculated directly in a cohort study as the ratio of the risk or incidence of the exposed to the unexposed group. However, in a case-comparison study the disease incidence in the exposed and unexposed population is unknown because the design begins with diseased cases and non-disease comparisons, not with exposed and unexposed groups. The question is not the cohort one of what is the probability that an event will occur in an exposed person, but what are the odds that a case was exposed? The RR should not therefore be estimated directly for case-comparison studies. Rather the odds should be estimated and the odds ratio used to infer the risk ratio, provided that:

- the comparisons are representative in terms of exposure of all people without the disease in the population from which the cases were drawn
- the cases are representative in terms of exposure of all people with the disease in the population from which the cases were drawn
- the cases are typical with respect to severity and diagnostic criteria.

Attributable risk

The final type of risk to be discussed here is **attributable risk**. This measure is used mainly in estimating the potential for prevention. In particular, it is used when assessing how much of the incidence can be prevented if the exposure is reduced to zero. Three measures of attributable risk are commonly used (Box 6.6):

- *Pure attributable risk (PAR)* represents the risk difference, or excess risk for the exposed population, and is calculated as a difference between the incidence rates for those exposed and unexposed groups.
- *Exposed attributable risk per cent (EAR%)* is when the difference between the risks is expressed as a percentage of the total risk experienced by the exposed group.
- *Population attributable risk per cent (PAR%)* is calculated as a difference between the incidence in the *total* population and the incidence in the unexposed as a ratio of the incidence of the *total* population.

Box 6.6 Measures of attributable risk

PAR = (Incidence for the exposed) − (Incidence for the unexposed)

$$EAR\% = \frac{(\text{Incidence for the exposed}) - (\text{Incidence for the unexposed})}{(\text{Incidence in exposed})} \times 100$$

$$PAR\% = \frac{(\text{Incidence for the total population}) - (\text{Incidence for the unexposed})}{(\text{Incidence in total population})} \times 100$$

Box 6.7 revisits the British doctor example. It can be seen that the relative risk for smoking is much higher for lung cancer than for coronary heart disease (CHD). This, however, does not necessarily mean that reducing smoking is going to have the greatest public health impact in terms of lives saved for lung cancer in comparison with CHD. The *attributable risk* for the case of lung cancer is (140 − 10) = 130. Of the total 140 deaths per 100,000 in smokers, 10 can be attributed to *background risk* (that is no smoking), so that 130 can be attributed as the maximum potential for prevention in the lung cancer case. For CHD mortality, although the relative risk is less, the attributable risk is greater. The background risk of no exposure is 413 and the exposed risk is 669 so the attributable risk, defined as the difference, is 256. The cessation of smoking would lead at maximum to a reduction of 130 lung cancer deaths per 100,000, but the equivalent figure for CHD would be nearly twice as great at 256. This results from the much greater baseline mortality level for CHD; heart disease is much more common than lung cancer.

For lung cancer, the EAR% is given by (140−10)/140 which equals 92 per cent, and for CHD equals (669−413)/669, that is 38 per cent. The measure is sometimes also known as the *attributable fraction* or *excess fraction*. The proportion of the lung cancer risk that can be attributed to

Box 6.7 Risk ratios and attributable risk, lung cancer and CHD mortality, British doctors

% Population attributable mortality risk	Age-adjusted death rates per 100,000		Attributable risk	% Exposed attributable risk	% Population attributable risk
	Smoker	Non-smoker			
Lung cancer	140	10	130	92	85
CHD	669	413	256	38	21

Note: The PAR% in the total population is based on 44 per cent of the population smoking.
Source: data from Doll and Peto 1976.

the exposure is 92 per cent while the equivalent figure for CHD is 38 per cent. The attributable risk percent is typically used as an indicator for the potential for prevention. In particular, the practising clinician is interested in the attributable risk for the exposed group, for example when giving a patient advice to stop smoking. This value gives the potential for prevention as it affects the exposed individual. The successful use of these measures depends on the relationship being truly causal, on the collection of unbiased measurements and on the sample, in this case British doctors, being suitable for generalization.

The important point to stress with the PAR% is that this value calculates the attributable risk for both smokers and non-smokers in the total population. The question now is not what is the effect of smoking cessation on the exposed group, but what is the overall effect on the wider community? In practice, we often do not know the incidence of the disease in the total population but we can derive it by knowing the proportion of the total population that is exposed, that is that smokes. For example, for the British doctors, the incidence rate of coronary heart disease among smokers is 669 per 100,000; and the incidence rate is 413 per 100,000 among non-smokers. Say we know from a national survey that some 44 per cent of the population smoke and 56 per cent do not. The incidence in the total population can then be calculated as a weighted average (Box 6.8). Thus 21.4 per cent of the incidence of CHD in the total population can be attributed to smoking. Therefore if smoking could be reduced to zero and the observed relation with smoking was causal then the maximum of the CHD deaths that could be prevented is 21.4 per cent.

In summary, the PAR% is of fundamental importance for public health policy and community preventative programmes. The PAR% puts the relative risk in the context of the whole population; it is generally a more useful index for assessing public health effects, whereas relative risk is useful for assessing the risk to an individual. Moreover as Gordis (1996: 160) reports, it is becoming of legal interest, for in the USA an attributable risk of 50 per cent might represent a quantitative determination of the legal definition of 'more likely than not' that a company has been responsible

---

Box 6.8   Calculating PAR%

$$\text{Population incidence} = \left(\text{Exposed incidence} \times \begin{array}{c}\text{Population}\\\text{proportion}\\\text{exposed}\end{array}\right) + \left(\text{Unexposed incidence} \times \begin{array}{c}\text{Proportion}\\\text{unexposed}\\\text{in population}\end{array}\right)$$

which in the CHD case gives:

$(669 \times 0.44) + (413 \times 0.56) = 525.6$ per 100,000

We can now put these values into the overall equation for the attributable risk in the total population:

$$\text{PAR\%} = \frac{525.6 - 413}{525.6} \times 100 = 0.214 \times 100 = 21.4$$

---

for environmental injury. Surprisingly, given its importance, the population attributable risk is reported much less frequently than the relative risk, but that may reflect epidemiology's tendency to use population data to focus on the individual and not on the population (see Chapters 7 and 8).

Risk and statistical inference

Just as a confidence interval was created in Chapter 3 for an SMR, so one can be created for relative risks and odds ratios. Formulae are given in Box 6.9 for the calculation of a confidence interval around the risk ratio and the odds ratio. The formulae used are conceptually the same as that used for the SMR, where a 95 per cent confidence 'buffer' is found by multiplying 1.96 (the number of standard errors which encompass 95 per cent of the values under a distribution of sample means) by the square root of the standard error and then adding and subtracting the exponential of this

---

Box 6.9   Confidence intervals for relative risk and odds ratios

A. *Confidence interval for relative risk*

(RR) exp $(\pm 1.96\sqrt{V})$

where $V = \dfrac{(1 - A)/(A + C)}{A} + \dfrac{(1 - B)/(B + D)}{B}$

B. *Confidence interval for odds ratio*

(OR) exp $\left(\pm 1.96\sqrt{(1/A) + (1/B) + (1/C) + (1/D)}\right)$

Note: exp (exponential) refers to the inverse of a natural log (ln).

---

value to and from the RR or OR value. In each example, it is the formulation of the standard error that is different. This natural log transformation is used because the sample distributions of relative risk and odds ratio are positively skewed. Taking a log transformation 'normalizes' the curve. For those unfamiliar with such transformations, the method can be seen as a mathematically based 'technical fix' to correct a skewed distribution to a bell-shaped distribution as described in the Appendix. The letters refer to the standard 2×2 table notation employed throughout this part of the book.

Analysing confounding

We have previously outlined how confounding by a third variable can bias the observed association between an exposure and an outcome variable. Our previous discussion was conceptual. Here the problem is extended and illustrated quantitatively using the 2×2 table. In particular, four hypothetical situations are provided which illustrate how confounding arises, and simultaneously show how stratification may be used to control for it and analyse its impact.

The example used is an examination of the association between the exposure of smoking and the outcome of CHD (McNeil 1996). Box 6.10 shows a stratified analysis whereby males and females are investigated separately (the first and second tables in each of A to D). The third table in each example represents an aggregate analysis of men and women together. If different results for the aggregate and stratified analysis are obtained, confounding is said to be taking place. In each of the 2×2 tables, CHD-y represents presence of disease, CHD-n represents absence of disease, S and NS represent exposure or not to smoking, respectively. Such tables could be derived from cohort, cross-sectional and case-comparison studies; consequently the degree of association between exposure and disease is measured by the odds ratio. The 2×2 tables that show the disaggregated results are known as *strata*.

The first example (A) shows the case where there is no confounding. There is an association between exposure and disease when the males and females are studied in isolation and when they are studied together. The stratification has shown the observed association is not due to a third variable – in this case sex – which has been 'controlled' via a subset analysis. In contrast, B shows a case of confounding. When the aggregated data for men and women are analysed there appears to be quite a strong relationship between the exposure and outcome with an odds ratio of 2.1. The stratified analysis, however, shows that this relationship is spurious; in each of the strata tables where sex is controlled there is no relationship between smoking and CHD (an odds ratio of 1). The apparent association disappears when the data are broken down by sex and the results suggest that the strength of the association between sex and CHD – when stratified by smoking status – should be explored.

In C the aggregate results indicate that there is no association between smoking and CHD, but when the two strata are analysed separately it is clear that there is a similar and marked association in each of the strata.

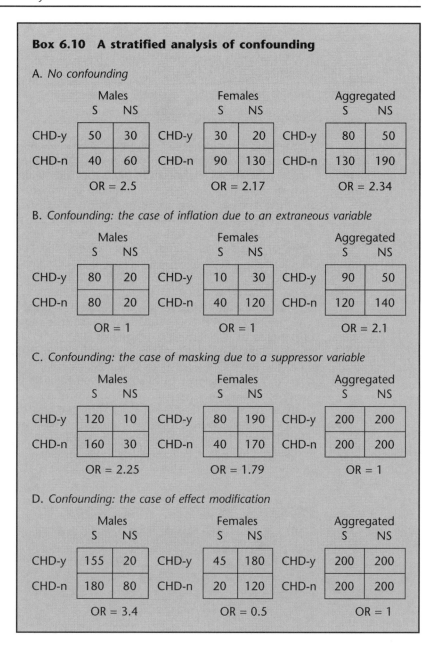

Box 6.10 A stratified analysis of confounding

A. *No confounding*

	Males				Females				Aggregated	
	S	NS			S	NS			S	NS
CHD-y	50	30		CHD-y	30	20		CHD-y	80	50
CHD-n	40	60		CHD-n	90	130		CHD-n	130	190
	OR = 2.5				OR = 2.17				OR = 2.34	

B. *Confounding: the case of inflation due to an extraneous variable*

	Males				Females				Aggregated	
	S	NS			S	NS			S	NS
CHD-y	80	20		CHD-y	10	30		CHD-y	90	50
CHD-n	80	20		CHD-n	40	120		CHD-n	120	140
	OR = 1				OR = 1				OR = 2.1	

C. *Confounding: the case of masking due to a suppressor variable*

	Males				Females				Aggregated	
	S	NS			S	NS			S	NS
CHD-y	120	10		CHD-y	80	190		CHD-y	200	200
CHD-n	160	30		CHD-n	40	170		CHD-n	200	200
	OR = 2.25				OR = 1.79				OR = 1	

D. *Confounding: the case of effect modification*

	Males				Females				Aggregated	
	S	NS			S	NS			S	NS
CHD-y	155	20		CHD-y	45	180		CHD-y	200	200
CHD-n	180	80		CHD-n	20	120		CHD-n	200	200
	OR = 3.4				OR = 0.5				OR = 1	

The third variable, sex, when not controlled has been suppressing or masking important associations. The separate association disappears completely when the data are pooled. In the fourth example (D), the aggregate relationship again shows an apparent lack of association between the exposure and the outcome, and this also changes when each strata is analysed separately. The difference now, however, is that there is a stronger association in one strata (males) than the other when sex is controlled. This case, where the odds ratios in the two subtables are markedly different, is known as effect modification. The third variable is interacting with exposure to modify the effect.

Beyond stratification analyses

Mantel and Haenszel (1959) proposed a rather more sophisticated set of methods for dealing with confounding in 2×2 tables. These methods are similar to stratified analysis in so far as they subdivide the data into strata. However, they go further and combine results to provide a composite measure of risk across groups of studies. This tests the association between two binary variables controlling for a stratification variable. We can use this method to look at different studies on the same topic, for example a series of aetiological studies of the relationship between smoking and lung cancer. Alternatively we can use it to combine results according to exposure and see, for example, whether different groups of patients respond similarly to different treatments. An example of this latter use is presented here as it will enable a further point of interest to be highlighted.

Consider a hypothetical study examining the responses of two groups of patients to two different treatments (Box 6.11). If the odds for treatments A and B are identical, the odds ratios would both be 1.0. For these data, the group 1 patients on treatment A are 1.6 times more likely to have a positive response to treatment than the group 1 patients on treatment B; while, for Group 2, those on treatment A are 3.2 times more likely to have a positive result than those on treatment B. Note that in this example the odds ratios are indicating risk of benefit not risk of an adverse event. It would appear that, for both patient groups, treatment A is effective in that it generates two odds ratios well in excess of 1. The question, however, is what the combined effect is across both patient

---

Box 6.11   Odds ratios: hypothetical treatment study

	Patient group A		Patient group B	
	Positive response	Negative response	Positive response	Negative response
Treatment A	14	28	16	32
Treatment B	9	29	7	45

The odds ratio for the patient group A:

$$\frac{14/28}{9/29} = 1.6$$

The odds ratio for the patient group B:

$$\frac{16/32}{7/45} = 3.2$$

groups – and, if we were dealing with smaller odds ratios, we would also want to consider whether, jointly, the two patient groups have a combined odds ratio greater than 1.

The Mantel–Haenszel statistic combines odds ratios across tables. The stratification variable in our example is the patient group. Box 6.12 shows how the statistic is calculated. Most computer packages for statistical analysis provide the required output. A statistical test of significance based on the chi-square statistic is also in common currency providing a confirmatory basis for assessing whether the observed Mantel–Haenszel statistic differs from one. For our example, the Mantel–Haenszel statistic is 2.277. We can treat this as a pooled odds ratio. It appears that large and confirmatory testing (not shown here) would generate a test statistic of 4.739 which would easily achieve significance and substantiate our view that treatment A has been more effective than treatment B for both groups of patients.

Box 6.12 Calculating the Mantel–Haenszel statistic

	Patient group A		Patient group B	
	Positive response	Negative response	Positive response	Negative response
Treatment A	14 (a)	28 (b)	16 (a)	32 (b)
Treatment B	9 (c)	29 (d)	7 (c)	45 (d)

Cell calculation	Group A	Group B	Row total	X/Y Mantel–Haenszel statistic
$\dfrac{ad}{a+b+c+d}$	5.1	7.2	12.3 (X)	2.277
$\dfrac{bc}{a+b+c+d}$	3.2	2.2	5.4 (Y)	

Moving beyond Mantel–Haenszel brings us to **modelling**. This topic is beyond the scope of this text. The essence of the approach is that it uses statistical theory to 'control by analysis'. Using ordinary least squares or, more normally with epidemiological data, logistic regression, the researcher attempts to build statistical models which 'explain' the variation in an outcome of interest in terms of a set of several exposure factors. For example, a model might seek to examine the respiratory function of a group of people in terms of their smoking status, their exposure to work-based pollutants, the amount of exercise they take, their age, their sex and so on. Output from the model-building process would indicate not only how good a model it is in terms of the individual and collective effectiveness of the exposure variables as determinants of the outcome data, but also the magnitude and direction of each identified effect. Thus we might learn that exposure A is more important than exposure B in determining outcome

C. More importantly, we would also know that the effect we attribute to exposure A is independent; the analysis is controlling for other effects.

Conclusion

This chapter has been able to present only a very basic overview of some of the more commonly used methods for epidemiological analysis. Our most detailed attention was reserved for the analysis of the 2×2 tables that are so common in epidemiological research. Fuller descriptions can be found in some of the excellent textbooks available on this subject (Box 6.13). Many other techniques, not described in this chapter, will also be found in these books.

Box 6.13 Further reading on epidemiological analysis

Abramson, J. (1994) *Making Sense of Data: A Self-instruction Manual on the Interpretation of Epidemiological Data*. Oxford: Oxford University Press.

Beaglehole, R., Bonita, R. and Kjellström, T. (1993) *Basic Epidemiology*. Geneva: World Health Organization.

Clayton, D. and Hills, M. (1993) *Statistical Models in Epidemiology*. Oxford: Oxford Science Publications.

Elwood, M. (1988) *Causal Relationships in Medicine: A Practical System for Critical Appraisal*. Oxford: Oxford University Press.

Friis, R. and Sellers, T. (1996) *Epidemiology for Public Health Practice*. Gaithersburg, MD: Aspen.

Greenberg, R., Daniels, S., Eley, J. and Boring, J. (1996) *Medical Epidemiology*. London: Prentice Hall International.

Hennekens, C. and Buring, J. (1987) *Epidemiology in Medicine*. Boston: Little Brown.

Kelsey, J., Whittemore, A., Evans, A. and Thompson, D. (1996) *Methods in Observational Epidemiology*. Oxford: Oxford University Press.

McNeil, D. (1996) *Epidemiological Research Methods*. Chichester: John Wiley.

Selvin, S. (1991) *Statistical Analysis of Epidemiologic Data*. Oxford: Oxford University Press.

Silman, A. (1995) *Epidemiological Studies: A Practical Guide*. Cambridge: Cambridge University Press.

Summary

- Most epidemiological studies involve presence/absence data: the relationship between exposure and outcome. A 2×2 table of disease status versus exposure can represent all such designs.

- An epidemiologist is usually interested in differential risks for different exposures; not absolute risk but *relative risk*. In essence, the relative risk is used to compare the incidence of a disease or condition in a group possessing a particular attribute or exposure with that in one without. The relative risk indicates the magnitude of the increased risk derived from the exposure.

- The population attributable risk per cent puts the relative risk in the context of the whole population; it is generally a more useful index for assessing public health effects, whereas relative risk is useful for assessing the risk to an individual.

- Stratification and the Mantel–Haenszel statistic provide a way to assess the impact of confounding within epidemiological studies.

Further reading

Beaglehole, R., Bonita, R. and Kjellström, T. (1993) *Basic Epidemiology,* Geneva: World Health Organization.
McNeil, D. (1996) *Epidemiological Research Methods.* Chichester: John Wiley.

Activities

1 Below are data obtained from a follow-up of the Health and Lifestyle Survey that relate to middle-aged men aged 41 to 60 in 1984, followed for some 13 years until 1997.

Total number of respondents   1224
Total number of deaths after follow-up   180

Use this information to calculate:

(a) the proportion dying, i.e. the absolute risk
(b) the equivalent estimate of the odds.

2 Examine the counts in the following examples. In each, the total of subjects (N = 100), the column marginals, and the row marginals are kept the same.
   Example 1 shows the case when the same proportion of the exposed as the unexposed are ill. In Example 2, however, all but one of the exposed have become ill, while all but one of the unexposed remain healthy. In Example 3 only one of the exposed becomes ill, while 49 of the unexposed report a diseased status.
   For each of these three different scenarios calculate the different RR and OR.

Example 1

		Exposure status		
		Yes	No	Total
Disease status	Yes	25	25	50
	No	25	25	50
		50	50	100

Example 2

		Exposure status		
		Yes	No	Total
Disease status	Yes	49	1	50
	No	1	49	50
		50	50	100

Example 3

		Exposure status		
		Yes	No	Total
Disease status	Yes	1	49	50
	No	49	1	50
		50	50	100

Try altering the counts systematically for yourself (but keeping the same fixed marginals) and observe how the risk ratio value alters. You can calculate the values easily with a hand calculator, but if you have access to the internet, point your browser to these websites that provide interactive calculations:

http://maddog.fammed.wisc.edu/~rbrown/epi.html
http://members.aol.com/johnp71/ctab2x2.html

All these sites give a lot more results from the 2 × 2 table than just the relative risk in the form of the risk ratio. Some of these other summary measures are considered later in the book.

3 Calculate the 95 per cent confidence interval around the relative risk for the following hypothetical data. (Remember first to calculate RR.)

	Not exposed	Exposed
Diseased	42	43
Not diseased	80	302

What does this confidence interval mean?

What does this result mean?

Repeat the process for the odds ratio in the following table:

	Exposed	Not exposed
Diseased	22	36
Not diseased	7	86

PART 2

ASSESSING AND APPLYING EPIDEMIOLOGY

PUTTING THE PARTS TOGETHER

In this chapter we present three case studies of epidemiology-related research. The reasons for doing this are threefold. First, and most simply, it
means that the application of some of the design and analysis techniques
covered in Part 1 can be illustrated in detail. Secondly, it allows us to
outline and show the use of a schema for critically appraising epidemiological research; this provides a useful prelude to the more detailed consideration of critical appraisal set out in the next chapter. Thirdly, it lets
us prompt you to begin thinking critically about epidemiological research
beyond 'simple' technical matters of design and analysis.

The studies covered have been selected because they illustrate the application of different research designs to the same problem and the insights,
explanations and accounts that result. They have, however, also been
chosen because they show clearly the strengths and weaknesses of epidemiological research in general and because they help stimulate critical
reflection about the whole process of epidemiology and reading epidemiology literature. The first case study focuses on scrutinizing research designs and analysis. It is therefore 'technically orientated'. The remaining
case studies involve a much broader and deeper consideration of epidemiology, health and medicine and society in general. More specifically, they
consider the issues of social and cultural biases and preconceptions prevalent in the social construction of disease.

After completing this chapter you should therefore be able to:

- demonstrate a practical understanding of the application of epidemiological design;
- be able to commence the qualitative evaluation of epidemiological research;
- show critical appreciation of this thing called epidemiology.

A schema for evaluating epidemiological research

Before presenting the case studies, it makes sense first to outline a generalized schema that can be used for evaluating any piece of epidemiological research. Later, this schema is applied in relation to some of the case study work. Chapter 8 contains consideration of more formal structured guidelines for critically appraising published epidemiological research. Elwood (1998) has developed the schema used in the present chapter and it is shown in Box 7.1.

In essence, Elwood's schema summarizes many of the issues outlined in Part 1. Thus many of the terms used should be familiar to you and you should be able to appreciate the relevance of many of the questions. Some parts will, however, be new to you and so we will quickly run through its structure and purpose. (If none of the schema makes any sense, you need to reread Part 1 now.)

The first part of the schema, section A, consists of five straightforward questions which seek to give a full description of the study's key characteristics. Although seemingly obvious, these questions are essential, and clear answers to each of them are vital – you need to be sure about what the study was doing and what was found in order to make a fair and accurate assessment of its quality. Sections B and C of the schema focus on internal validity. As noted earlier, internal validity can be defined as 'a measure of how easily a difference in outcome between two groups can be attributed to the effects of the exposure or intervention' (Elwood 1998: 59). As such, therefore, this aspect of validity relates to the adequacy of the workings of the study (making it 'internal'), and it focuses on design and analysis issues. In section B, one key aspect of validity is considered: non-causal explanations. These are mechanisms that would produce the results but which do not relate to an actual causal process. There are three of these, all of which you have encountered before: bias, confounding and chance. Section C considers the other key aspect of internal validity: the positive features of causation. If our result is not produced by non-causal mechanisms, what counts as positive indicators of causality? There are five main indicators (Box 7.2). Many of these coincide with those laid out in another well known schema often used for assessing epidemiological research, that of Austin Bradford-Hill (Hill 1965).

The fourth part, section D, covers the other dimension of validity: external validity. This is concerned with 'the way in which the results of a study can be generalised to a wider population' (Elwood 1998: 60). Thus, if we believe genuine causal processes have produced our results, to whom do they apply? As can be seen, Elwood's schema considers this in terms of three specific populations. The **eligible population** is those

> **Box 7.1 Elwood's schema for assessing epidemiological research**
>
> A. *Description of the evidence*
>   1 Exposure or intervention: what was the intervention or exposure?
>   2 Outcome: what was the outcome?
>   3 Study design: what was the study design?
>   4 Study population: what was the study population?
>   5 Main result: what was the main result?
>
> B. *Internal validity – consideration of non-causal explanations*
>   6 Observation bias: are the results likely to be affected by observation bias?
>   7 Confounding: are the results likely to be affected by confounding?
>   8 Chance: are the results likely to be affected by chance variation?
>
> C. *Internal validity – consideration of positive features of causation*
>   9 Time: is there a correct time relationship?
>   10 Strength: is the relationship strong?
>   11 Dose–response: is there a dose–response relationship?
>   12 Consistency: are the results consistent within the study?
>   13 Specificity: is there any specificity within the study?
>
> D. *External validity – generalization of the results*
>   14 Eligible population: can the study results be applied to the eligible population?
>   15 Source population: can the results be applied to the source population?
>   16 Other populations: can the results be applied to other relevant populations?
>
> E. *Comparison of the results with other evidence*
>   17 Consistency: are the results consistent with other evidence, particularly evidence from studies of similar or more powerful study designs?
>   18 Specificity: does the total evidence suggest any specificity?
>   19 Plausibility: are the results plausible, in terms of a biological mechanism?
>   20 If a major effect is shown, is it coherent with the distribution of the exposure and the outcome?
>
> *Source*: Elwood 1998.

people who are defined (on the basis of explicit criteria) as being eligible for entry into the study (the actual people in the study – the participants – are obviously a subset of these). The *source population* is the broader, more generally defined population from which the eligible population is drawn. The **target population** is the population to which the results

Box 7.2 Positive indicators of causality

- *Time*: for a factor or process to be causal we must be certain that it preceded the event and not vice versa (the latter being 'reverse causation' – see Chapter 4).
- *Strength*: a stronger relationship, that is a larger relative risk, is more likely to reflect a causal relationship. (It should be noted, however, that true causal factors can produce only small increases in risk especially where they are only one of a number operating at the same time. If widely distributed through a population, factors with small effects may be more significant in terms of public health than rarer, larger exposures.)
- *Dose–response*: if the effect of an exposure increases (or decreases, if preventative) in proportion to its dose then this does suggest it is causal. (It should be noted, however, that there can be threshold or all-or-none effects.)
- *Consistency*: associations should be seen across a wide range of subjects within the study. (If this does not hold, it suggests that the hypothesis of causation can be specified more precisely.)
- *Specificity*: if there is a specific association between one causal factor and one outcome it is sometimes considered as good evidence of causality. This criterion is, however, problematic and is rarely an absolute, especially nowadays in the age of chronic degenerative rather than infectious conditions.

can be applied (unlike the others this is not fixed or determined by the study itself). To illustrate these notions, we can think of a study of an exposure to a particular dangerous chemical in a particular factory. The eligible population could be those who work directly with the chemical (importantly, this will include those who agree to participate and those who do not – there should not be any differences between these groups); the source population would be all workers in the factory; the target population would include all other factories where this chemical is used or, indeed, any other place it is encountered. While thinking of external validity in terms of these specific populations is appropriate, it can also be thought of more broadly especially with regard to experimental and intervention studies; for example, are the doses/exposures/routes of transmission in experimental settings similar to those in the real world?

The fifth and final part, section E, focuses on comparing a study's results with pre-existing evidence. Attention here again extends beyond the internal workings of the study and centres on whether the results are:

- Consistent: have they been found elsewhere?
- Specific: do they apply to specific outcomes and not others and is this as hypothesized?

- Biologically plausible: do they make biological sense? Obviously, this needs to be applied carefully otherwise we would have no new knowledge.
- Coherent: do they fit with what is known about the (broader) distribution of both the exposure and the outcome?

Case study I: childhood cancer and the nuclear industry

The first case study considers a range of published epidemiological literature relating to the possible adverse health effects to children associated with the Sellafield nuclear reprocessing plant in Cumbria, England. We begin by charting some of the background to this work and some of the initial investigations. We then go on to apply the schema just outlined to some of the later, more important, studies.

Opened in 1947, and commencing full operations in 1950, Sellafield (or Windscale and Calder Hall as it was first known) attracted attention in the early 1980s after the screening of a television documentary describing a cluster of leukaemia cases amongst young people near the plant. In particular, it was suggested that there was a tenfold excess within the village of Seascale, three kilometres to the south of the plant. We must at this point emphasize that, although seeming large in absolute terms, this excess only consisted of a small number of cases, as leukaemia is a rare disease. As will be seen, this rareness quality has considerable bearing on the design and analysis of all the subsequent work. An independent government enquiry soon followed which, drawing on local routine health statistics, confirmed the cluster and recommended a series of further epidemiological studies be conducted and a group of experts be commissioned to review and judge the evidence as and when it became available (Black 1984).

Following a typical sequence of epidemiological investigation, attention was first directed at substantiating the peculiarity of the cluster and that it did, indeed, represent an excess of cases. Detailed and geographically extensive descriptive epidemiological work was conducted. More specifically, an analysis of childhood cancer by small area (electoral wards) across the entire Northern Regional Health Authority (RHA) area was carried out (Craft *et al.* 1984, 1993; Openshaw *et al.* 1988). While we will not cover the exact methods used in this work, the rationale was similar to that described for death rates (Chapter 2). Thus, the number of cases that would be expected in an area given its population size and structure was compared with the observed number of cases; observed–expected differences were then tested to see whether they were likely to have occurred by chance. For interest, we can note that in work like this, expected numbers are not calculated using a standard population as with death rates but are based on a well known statistical distribution, the **Poisson distribution** (see Kirkwood 1988: chapter 17), that describes the occurrence of rare events following a random, rather than systematic and causal, process.

This descriptive work suggested that the cluster around Sellafield did indeed represent more cases than would be expected by chance and that

Seascale had, in a statistical sense, the most extreme rate of childhood leukaemia of all the 675 small areas constituting the Northern RHA. While such work usefully completed the 'distribution picture', it obviously said little about the 'determinants question' (Chapter 1). Thus, as well as recommending further descriptive work, the inquiry also explicitly requested studies based on the analytical observational designs outlined earlier: that is, cohort and case-comparison studies. The causal thinking that was framing these subsequent investigations was clear. As proposed by the television documentary, the primary hypothesis was that the excess of cases was caused by a general environmental effect. That is, living near Sellafield led to exposure to radiation, a known carcinogen linked particularly to leukaemia. This exposure was due to discharges from the plant either in the sea or in the air. Thus, the leading causal hypothesis centred on non-specific environmental contamination. As we will see, evidence from the epidemiological studies turned out to support a quite different interpretation.

The Sellafield cohort studies

The first analytical, observational work published consisted of two cohort studies by Gardner and his colleagues at the Medical Research Council's Environmental Epidemiology Unit at the University of Southampton (Gardner *et al.* 1987a, b). One of these dealt with a schools cohort – children born since 1950 who attended schools in Seascale up until 1983 – whilst another considered a birth cohort – children who were actually born in Seascale between 1950 and 1983. The purpose of these studies was twofold: first, to confirm more conclusively the excess of leukaemia cases given the recognized weaknesses of the earlier descriptive work (the main one being that it had given little or no direct information on the individuals with or without the disease); secondly, to throw some light on what may be causing it; more specifically, given the cohorts studied, did the causal process operate before birth/early in life or did it operate later in life (from school age onwards)? Since both studies were identical in terms of design and analysis apart from the actual cohort under study, we will only carry out an appraisal of one of them, the birth cohort (Gardner *et al.* 1987b), in light of Elwood's schema.

Description of the evidence

The objective was to assess the effect of a specific exposure: being born in Seascale, West Cumbria (that is, in close proximity to Sellafield). The main outcome measure is death from leukaemia, although cases of other cancers are also considered. The study design was a retrospective (historical) cohort study: the study population was identified through past and current birth, health, electoral and school registers. Rather than explicitly or implicitly gathering together a non-exposed series, the exposed cohort was compared with expected numbers based on national mortality statistics. To avoid small numbers (leukaemia being a rare disease), the study covers a period of 33 years. The main result is that there is an excess of leukaemia cases: over the period 1950–83 there are five deaths compared with 0.53 expected from death rates in England and Wales. This tenfold difference seems to suggest a strong relationship between place of exposure and death.

Internal validity – non-causal explanations

Whilst there is always a strong chance of observation (recall) bias in any retrospective design, it would seem to have been minimized in the Sellafield birth cohort study owing to a reliance on official ('objective') sources of information. Since multiple sources are used – a variety of official registers – this allows **triangulation** (comparison) between them, thus further reducing the chance of any bias as well as ensuring more complete coverage. At the same time, using a 'person-years method' reduces measurement bias. This considers each cohort member in terms of the number of years they were resident in Seascale and ensures that the high levels of mobility identified among Seascale residents do not adversely affect any calculations.

In terms of confounding, the expected number of deaths is standardized for age and sex, thus taking account of both of these possible confounders. Few other variables, however, are taken into account and one particularly problematic possibility is that the social class distribution in Seascale is rather different from that across the rest of the country. More specifically, children from higher social class families are considerably over-represented in the Seascale population and high social class has been associated with higher rates of leukaemia in other work. Thus, following the definition given in Chapter 4, this is certainly a potential confounder as it is associated with both the exposure and the outcome measure. The authors claim, however, drawing on previous descriptive work on childhood cancer in the north west of England, that leukaemia cases in that part of the country do not have a different social class distribution from those in the population as a whole. The possibility of the excess deaths being due to chance is taken into account by presenting confidence intervals for the observed/expected ratio (based on the Poisson distribution). It is immediately apparent, therefore, whether any ratio is statistically significantly different from the value (1) of no difference.

Internal validity – positive features of causation

Since we are dealing with a cohort study based on a series of births with the exposure being place of birth, it is certain that the exposure preceded the outcome. Although, strictly speaking, no actual relative risk values are produced in this type of cohort study, the strength of association can be assessed by the ratio of observed to expected deaths from leukaemia: 5 actual deaths compared with 0.53 expected. While pseudo-analyses of a **dose–response relationship** are presented (Gardner *et al.* 1987b: table VII) this issue is not considered in detail and no analyses are reported stratified according to years of residence in Seascale. This is understandable given that such information is very hard to obtain at least to any reasonable degree of accuracy. Given such a small number of outcome events, it is also difficult to say much about consistency. In terms of specificity, the results are certainly strongest for leukaemia though excess deaths are also found for other types of cancer; deficits are found for other conditions (stillbirths, infant mortality) and this may be significant.

External validity

Results would appear to be generalizable with the participant and source population since in a study like this, where coverage seems to be very high (not least because of the considerable efforts taken to identify all births), they are all basically the same. Those who participated were those who were eligible, who were those in the source population. The generalization to other populations is more complex. Is Sellafield and its surrounding environment the same as other nuclear installations? Are English children the same as other children? Similar studies based on other installations in other countries are obviously relevant here.

Comparison with other evidence

Studies of rare diseases are always difficult given the small numbers involved and so, in light of this, consistency with other studies is crucial. Excesses have been found around other British nuclear installations, although it is only around Sellafield and Dounreay that they were large. What is of most relevance here, however, is that similar results were not found in the other cohort: an excess of deaths from leukaemia was not found amongst children attending schools in Seascale (Gardner *et al.* 1987a). Thus, there would seem to be a specific relationship suggesting that the exposure was uniquely associated with pre- or early life. In terms of biological plausibility there is evidence showing connections between radiation and leukaemia. Since, however, the exposure considered in this study was very broadly defined (living near Sellafield), precise biological mechanisms are not so relevant.

The Sellafield case-comparison study

While useful, the cohort studies remained rather vague about the precise causal process(es) involved in the apparent excess of childhood leukaemia cases in Seascale. By considering exposure in terms of either 'being born in' or 'being schooled in' Seascale, little could be said about what exactly was causing the excess cases. In fairness, it should be acknowledged this was not actually the main purpose of the cohort studies: they were intended mainly to confirm the excess suggested by the earlier and more simple descriptive work. Nevertheless, it remained the case that little was known about causal mechanisms and a study was needed which focused on examining individual factors characterizing cases. This work took the form of a case-comparison study and was again conducted by Gardner and colleagues (Gardner *et al.* 1990a, b).

   As you have seen the schema applied once before, this time we will simply provide a summary. This is given in Box 7.3. It should be apparent

Box 7.3   **A summary assessment of Gardner *et al.*'s (1990a)**
Sellafield case-comparison study

A. *Description of evidence*

1 Exposure	Antenatal X-rays, viral infections, social class, behaviours, proximity to plant, parental employment in plant, parental radiation doses
2 Outcome	Leukaemia, non-Hodgkin's lymphoma, Hodgkin's disease
3 Design	Case-control study (matched)
4 Study population	Cases: 97 cases of the three diseases (52 with leukaemia) controls: two sets of controls, one with mother living in West Cumbria the other with mother living in same parish as case; N = 1001 in total
5 Main result	Relative risks particularly high for paternal employment at Sellafield, 2.44 (95%: 1.04, 5.71), and paternal radiation doses (>100 mSv) before child's conception, 6.42 (95%: 1.57, 26.3)

B. *Non-causal explanations*

6 Observation bias	Possible given retrospective design, especially for some antenatal factors, though multiple sources used and high concordance/low bias reported
7 Confounding	Age and sex controlled for by matching (also place of residence for local controls); analyses conditional on other risk factors
8 Chance	Confidence intervals presented

C. *Features consistent with causation*

9 Time	Uncertain for various exposures but presumably OK for paternal exposures (i.e. before birth)
10 Strength	Strong association for certain exposures but large confidence intervals emphasize based on small numbers
11 Dose–response	Seen for radiation dose before six months but not for total dose
12 Consistency	Information not available
13 Specificity	Information not available

D. *External validity*

14 Eligible popn	All cases from 1950 to 1985 included
15 Source popn	Same as eligible
16 Other popn	If causal pathway is radiation exposure, then potentially widely applicable

E. *Comparison with other evidence*

17 Consistency	Few other similar detailed studies at time of publication or now

18 Specificity effects	Greatest for leukaemia though significant also for non-Hodgkin's lymphoma
19 Plausibility	Evidence from X-rays and some animal experiments lend credence, but H bomb survivors do not
20 Coherence	Difficult to establish as rare exposure/outcome but some discrepancies with work around other nuclear installations and similarly exposed groups

this later work was, for the most part, well designed, carefully carried out and appropriately analysed. It should also be apparent that it suggested a very different causal explanation from that which dominated original thinking. Rather than there being a general environmental effect, the case-comparison study's findings suggested the causal pathway was specifically connected with paternal exposure to radiation, particularly in the period immediately prior to conception. Although not unchallenged, this finding does demonstrate the potential power, and central place, of observational epidemiological research.

The story that we have told here has a significant postscript. Perhaps unsurprisingly given the findings of the case-comparison study, a number of personal injury lawsuits were subsequently issued against British Nuclear Fuels (BNF), the company running Sellafield, by families of some of the cases. Following a long and exhaustive trial process, details of which can be found in Wakeford (1998), the presiding judge found in favour of BNF in two of these cases thus, in effect, refuting the 'Gardner hypothesis' of paternal exposure. Significantly, the judge did not find fault with the work (in fact, he is on record as describing Gardner et al.'s case-control study as 'a good study, well carried out and presented' (Wakeford 1998: 322)). Nor did he dispute that there was an excess of cases. Rather, he believed that the causal pathway suggested by the case-control study's findings did not stand up when 'viewed within the broad context of scientific evidence' (Wakeford 1998: 322). As Doll et al. (1994) put it (though obviously this was disputed by Gardner himself), the parental radiation exposure thesis lacked biological plausibility given what is known about radiation genetics and the heritability of childhood leukaemia, especially in light of estimated levels of doses at Sellafield. Also, it did not cohere with what was found in relation to other, similarly exposed groups in similar situations.

Given this outcome, three key points can be made. First, perhaps more than anything else this ending underlines how certainty is a scarce resource when working with epidemiological evidence. In many ways this arises because epidemiologists are often denied the use of experimental designs. Saying this, however, experiments themselves are not without problems, making it best, perhaps, to think of 'appropriate methodologies' (McKinlay 1993) rather than 'gold standards'. Secondly, therefore, it should be apparent that any epidemiological evidence needs to be subjected to careful, critical appraisal, regardless of the research design on which it is based. It is for this reason that the schema of Elwood that has been outlined and used here is extremely valuable and it is also the rationale for the more formal discussion of critical appraisal in the next chapter. Thirdly, and finally, the judge's decision (which was, incidentally, supported by the expert committee mentioned above (Committee on Medical Aspects of Radiation in the Environment 1996)) reveals how judgements about epidemiological evidence are often made not only in light of a study's internal formulation and workings but also in terms of how the study's findings relate to the external world and other bodies of evidence.

Case study II: the confounding of occupation and smoking

For our second case study we consider a small body of research which focuses on one of the potential major problems facing epidemiological research: confounding. This work has been chosen because it provides a useful bridge from the Sellafield studies to our final case study. So far, confounding has been presented as a technical issue – something which reduces internal validity – and, indeed, our whole discussion of Sellafield remained extremely technically orientated. By technical we mean that we concentrated on issues of an applied, practical nature relating mostly to study design, analysis and existing bodies of evidence. Put another way, we concentrated on the mechanics, or the 'nitty-gritty' of what was done, how it was done and how it related to what had been done previously. As we now show, although confounding is certainly a technical issue, it can also be thought of as indicating bias and error that arises from social, political and cultural processes. The second case study, and that which follows, provides an opportunity to think more broadly and deeply about epidemiology, health and medicine as a whole.

Smoking and occupation

Smoking is widely recognized as a major cause of lung disease and other conditions. As such, it has come to be seen as one of the major contributory factors to workers' ill health. At the same time, and following from this, it is widely recognized that if researchers are to uncover the other dangers to which workers are exposed, they must 'control for' workers' tobacco consumption. In short, smoking is regarded as a potentially major confounder in studies of occupational health: it is associated with certain workers in certain occupations and it is also associated with disease. By failing to recognize this, the effects of smoking are likely to be taken inappropriately for the effects of other occupational exposures; in other words, the latter will be overestimated.

Some epidemiological research has, however, suggested that we need to think even more carefully about the confounding between smoking and occupation. Put briefly, rather than seeing smoking as exaggerating the effects of working, working may have exaggerated how we perceive the effects of smoking. Alternatively, as the main researcher in this area has put it, 'does smoking kill workers, or does working kill smokers?' (Sterling 1978). In both cases, confounding is implied but obviously what is given priority in causal terms is very different between the two. Furthermore, we are much more likely to think of the former rather than the latter: thus, smoking is more likely to be thought of as a confounder of working which serves to exaggerate its effects, rather than working being thought of as a confounder of smoking which exaggerates its effects.

We will now consider some of the relevant research. To start, our approach will very much be a technical one and we will use some of the ideas and criteria contained within Elwood's schema. After this, however, we will take a broader approach as we try to tackle the question of why smoking tends to be given greater causal priority and why working is rarely seen as exaggerating its effects. As you will see, this will lead us to certain social and cultural biases, rather than simply technical ones.

Descriptive epidemiologies

A North American researcher, Theodore Sterling, has conducted most of the work on the confounding of smoking and occupation. First, and most simply, Sterling observes that many occupational health studies have in fact shown that occupation and not smoking is the major cause of lung cancer: a list and discussion of many of these are given in Sterling (1978). Secondly, Sterling argues that studies identifying smoking as the major cause of occupational lung disease are seriously flawed. For the most part, this arises from a particular instance of information bias. To demonstrate this, let us consider Table 7.1. This table, drawn up from a close detailed analysis of occupational status based on one of the few data sources with sufficient information, shows three key smoking risks for two groups of workers: those who would tend to be exposed to toxic fumes and dusts ('blue collar') and those who would not ('professional').

Table 7.1 shows clearly that smoking risk is substantially highest amongst the group with the greatest exposure to workplace hazards; thus, as the authors put it, 'the category of smoker in a statistical sense is an index of likelihood of exposure to occupational hazards' (Sterling and Weinkam 1990: 461). Unfortunately, however, as Sterling and colleagues outline, most epidemiological studies that try to deal with this do so inadequately as they use extremely imprecise measures of occupational exposure such as social class. Thus, information bias occurs since the two confounding variables are rarely measured with the same degree of accuracy or completeness.

There are other threats to the internal validity of much of the research considering the relative significance of smoking and occupation. Chief amongst these is the use of inappropriate comparison groups when calculating SMRs and other measures of smoking-related disease incidence. Sterling and Weinkam (1990) draw particular attention to one instance of this 'healthy worker effect'. As they state, most studies have worked with SMRs standardized for the general population; given that this group is always less healthy than the working population as it includes

Table 7.1 Smoking risk by occupational group

Smoking habits	Blue collar (%)	Professional (%)
Amount smoked		
20+	48.4	7.2
10–19	49.5	7.8
1–9	40.8	9.5
None	38.3	15.7
Smoking status		
Never smoked	37.7	16.8
Former smoker	38.9	14.6
Age started		
Younger than 20	48.9	7.5
20+	39.0	12.0

Source: Sterling and Weinkam 1990: 460.

those unfit to work, occupational exposures are underestimated in them-selves, and by extension, in relation to smoking. One remaining weak-ness is that many studies simply fail to recognize the confounding of smoking and occupation. Sterling and Weinkam (1990) outline the case of bladder cancer and show that researchers are much more likely to calculate the risk of the disease with respect to smoking than for occupa-tion and few calculate estimates of the effect of smoking independent of occupation.

In the foregoing we have presented important evidence relating to the confounding of smoking and occupation such that the effects of the latter are likely to be underestimated while the effects of the former will be exaggerated. So far, however, we have said little about what the size of these distortions may be. Work by British researchers has, however, tried to address this question. Using data from the Whitehall study – a longi-tudinal study of British civil servants – Davey-Smith and Shipley (1991) calculate age-adjusted mortality risks according to both employment grade and smoking status. They go on to calculate the number of deaths that would be avoided if smokers either stopped smoking or had never started smoking. First, they do this assuming that the level of risk drops to that within the cohort overall; next, they do it assuming it drops to the level specific to the employment grade. The difference between these can be taken as an estimate of the confounding of smoking and occupation on mortality risk and it is found to be approximately 30 per cent. As the authors state, this 'demonstrates the importance of such confounding'; at the same time, they also believe that, if anything, their work underesti-mates it (Davey-Smith and Shipley 1991: 1299).

From technical to cultural

Taking a technical approach, it can be seen that the confounding of smoking and occupation can be expected to be a very real problem in epidemiological research. Having got this far, however, you may well be thinking that it is not necessarily an insurmountable problem and that it is one that can be handled if the codes of good practice laid out in Chapters 4 are followed and adhered to. While we would agree with this to some extent, we would also suggest that technical answers are not wholly sufficient as the confounding of occupation and smoking is not simply a technical issue but also a social, cultural and political one.

Reading the work of Sterling and others, it is striking how many undoubtedly competent, intelligent, gifted epidemiological researchers fail to explore and consider the confounding of smoking and occupation. Since it is hard to believe that they are not aware of confounding, it suggests there is a deeply held and longstanding cultural bias against explanations focusing on work conditions as opposed to individual behaviours (see Doyal and Epstein 1983). At times, this bias is clearly visible. Perhaps the most obvious manifestation of it can be seen when we consider which information is deemed worthy of being routinely collected. As Sterling (1978) points out, cancer registries in Canada and the USA always gather information about smoking but never about occupation. Although simple, this example usefully flags up the limitations of technical solutions: if the 'relevant' data are not there, there is little point in having well specified, technically sophisticated statistical models.

Perhaps more significantly, however, it is not simply a case of what we choose to measure and what we choose not to. Often, how we do the very measuring is shaped by cultural assumptions. Drawing on Sterling once again, he reports strong evidence of a diagnostic bias in lung cancer cases: asbestos workers who smoke are much more likely to be given a diagnosis of lung cancer whilst non-smoking asbestos workers are more likely to be given a diagnosis of cancer from some site other than the lung. (For other examples of sociocultural assumptions shaping health data see Prior 1985; Bloor et al. 1987; McKinlay 1996). Again, this underlines the limitations of a purely technical approach: even where 'relevant' data are available, they may exhibit certain cultural assumptions and priorities in ways which cannot readily be taken into account whatever study designs or statistical methods are applied.

One other aspect of this cultural bias is the way in which the work of Sterling and others has been resolutely ignored by most epidemiologists. Few workers refer to or cite Sterling's work despite its considerable implications. Sterling and Weinkam account for this in three ways. First, epidemiologists are part of the advantaged 'investigating classes' and so are indifferent to those in less advantaged 'blue collar' occupations. Secondly, the dominant cultural attitude within more advantaged sections of society is that health is a matter of personal, individual responsibility with individuals being free to choose either to live healthy lives or not: from this position, disease is very much seen as punishment for wrong-doing. Thirdly, epidemiologists are especially likely to belong to groups that campaign against smoking (presumably as this fits closely with the perspective just outlined). In light of this, they are not neutral, disinterested observers – our usual view of scientists and experts – but people with specific positions, perspectives and interests.

Case study III: respiratory disease and the North American mining industry

In our third case study, we wish to illustrate further one of the important ideas just raised: that is, how the way in which disease is recognized, classified and recorded is often an intrinsically social/cultural and, by implication, political process. Our example focuses on respiratory disease within part of the American mining industry (Smith 1981). There are, however, close parallels with events in the UK as evidenced by the large compensation claims awarded to British miners in March 1999.

It is now well recognized that working underground in the mining industry is a dangerous and unhealthy occupation. A detailed historical analysis of the Pennsylvanian coalfields in North America emphasizes, however, the way in which the disease implications of mining are often the subject of socially and historically specific interpretations and classifications. In this particular case, four distinct phases can be recognized each of which sustains a particular **social construction** of miners' disease experiences relating to the prevailing economic, social and political circumstances.

In the first instance, as the coalfields were being established, miners organized their own health care through mutual aid associations. At this time, it was increasingly recognized that working underground produced respiratory problems from breathing gas and dust. As the coalfield grew and became more profitable, however, the owners of the mines and their companies assumed responsibility for the miners' health care. Following this, although specific conditions were recognized, it was no longer acknowledged that working underground was generally harmful for respiratory health and illness was increasingly viewed as a product of the miners' lifestyle, particularly their alcohol consumption.

This reluctance to recognize miners' respiratory disease as an occupationally related condition – black lung – prevailed until relatively recently despite evidence from a number of doctors (usually employed by the miners' union) to the contrary. In the 1960s, however, retiring miners, aware of the industry's prosperity, began a campaign for compensation. After a number of protests, this was agreed but only on the basis of a specific clinical diagnosis – coal miner's pneumoconiosis – which had to come from X-ray evidence. In short, to win compensation the lungs of a miner had to show visibly evident pathological changes.

Unsurprisingly, this extremely narrow and precise disease construction did not satisfy the miners. For one thing, many were excluded despite being severely disabled because their disease could not be confirmed by X-ray; others with little disability but positive X-rays, meanwhile, were included. Overall, the numbers qualifying were extremely low, given the very specific criteria. In light of this, further protests were organized with the intention of redefining the disease not in terms of specific, and hence individualized, diagnostic criteria but as a general illness and disability produced by the total workplace environment. Despite some setbacks, laws were finally passed at the end of the 1970s in accordance with this so that ex-miners who had worked underground for a long time received compensation.

From this review, it should be apparent that disease is not necessarily a simple, unproblematic biological entity. Instead, it is often a complex, contested social and cultural construction. In the example we have considered, it is important to stress that it was not better or more accurate technical knowledge that led to the disease being defined differently in different time periods. Instead, it was a process of social and political struggle in which all those involved were positioned according to certain interests and certain configurations of power and influence. As this example might be considered to be a rather obvious and extreme one, we should just quickly note that much less seemingly contentious conditions such as diabetes and hypertension are far from being clear-cut and easily defined. In light of all of this, therefore, epidemiologists need to consider who defines disease, and in whose interest. Furthermore, when doing this, they need to recognize that the process of defining disease is likely to be socially, culturally and geographically specific.

Conclusion

This chapter has examined the research designs and methodologies used in three epidemiological case studies concerned with occupational exposures to disease. The approach taken in the first case study was technically orientated, whilst the two other involved a much broader and deeper consideration of epidemiology. It is hoped that this chapter has also helped to develop an awareness that all epidemiological research occurs within broader social, cultural and political contexts. In doing so we have not meant to take the ground away from under the epidemiologist's feet. In principle, there is nothing wrong with the design and analysis techniques covered in Chapters 4 and 5 and they are very useful in helping to answer particular questions (Chapter 8). Such techniques are, however, always applied by somebody, somewhere, and that can make a difference. Moreover, they represent one type of 'account' or 'way of knowing' about health, disease and illness (see also Chapter 9). Seen in this way, therefore, the epidemiological methods reviewed here are certainly not worthless, but their use does require care, attention and reflection.

Summary

- Epidemiological research requires thinking beyond 'simple' technical matters of design and analysis and appreciating the broader social, cultural and political context in which epidemiology is located.

- Elwood's schema provides themes on which to focus when assessing epidemiological studies: the study's key characteristics in terms of aims, background, methods and conclusions; its internal validity; its external validity and its relationship to existing work.

Further reading

Elwood, J. (1998) *Critical Appraisal of Epidemiological Studies and Clinical Trials*. Oxford: Oxford University Press.

Pearce, N. (1996) Traditional epidemiology, modern epidemiology, and public health, *American Journal of Public Health*, 86: 678–83.

Sterling, T. and Weinkam, J. (1990) The confounding of occupation and smoking and its consequences, *Social Science and Medicine*, 30: 457–67.

Wakeford, R. (1998) Epidemiology and litigation – the Sellafield childhood leukaemia cases, *Journal of the Royal Statistical Society Series A*, 161: 313–25.

Activities

1 On the basis of Elwood's schema and what you have read in Part 1, try answering the following questions.

   (a) Are experimental designs stronger on internal validity or on external validity, or neither?

   (b) Are observational designs stronger on internal validity or on external validity, or neither?

   (c) Which is more important, internal validity or external validity?

   (d) Is it possible to have high internal validity and high external validity or are they in some sense mutually exclusive?

2 The text presents a summary of some important studies of the health implications of the nuclear industry. Read the papers for yourself. The references are:

Gardner, M.J., Hall, A.J., Downs, S. and Terrell, J.D. (1987) Follow up study of children born to mothers resident in Seascale, West Cumbria (birth cohort), *British Medical Journal*, 295, 822–7.

Gardner, M.J., Snee, M.P., Hall, A.J., Powell, C.A., Downs, S. and Terrell, J.D. (1990) Results of case-control study of leukaemia and lymphoma among young people near the Sellafield nuclear plant in West Cumbria, *British Medical Journal*, 300, 423–9.

Gardner, M.J., Hall, A.J., Snee, M.P., Downs, S., Powell, C.A. and Terrell, J.D. (1990) Methods and basic data of case-control study of leukaemia and lymphoma among young people near the Sellafield nuclear plant in West Cumbria, *British Medical Journal*, 300, 429–34.

3 Thinking of your own work as a health professional, are there any diseases which you regularly encounter which are defined in different ways by different groups in society? What are the implications deriving from each definition?

EVIDENCE-BASED HEALTH CARE

Much of the recent interest in epidemiology has focused on its application to the development of **evidence-based health care**. Evidence-based health care (EBHC) is concerned with the identification of the best and most appropriate ways of treating and managing patients. It is full of jargon and buzzwords such as clinical effectiveness, systematic reviews, **critical appraisal** skills, meta-analysis, numbers needed to treat (or harm) and so forth. In this chapter we unpack this jargon and provide a brief introduction to the skills, methods and techniques required to practice evidence-based health care.

By the end of the chapter, you should:

- have an appreciation of the impetus behind the emergence of evidence-based health care;
- understand the centrality of epidemiological evidence to evidence-based health care;
- grasp the basic techniques applied in the practice of evidence-based health care.

The next section briefly considers the case for evidence-based health care. The rest of the chapter discusses how we can find, manage and make sense of health-based research. There are sections that consider different types of evidence, literature searching, systematic reviews, meta-analysis and critical reading and appraisal.

Background

There are numerous examples of unproven and ineffective medical treatments. Some drugs and therapies can do more harm than good even when allowance is made for the great variation in medical practices among different doctors and health professionals (Cochrane 1972). Some medicines and treatments have never been tested using clinical trials (antibiotics being a notable example) and to do so now would be unethical as we know about their efficacy. What is lacking is sound information on **clinical effectiveness**. What do we mean by clinical effectiveness? Li Wan Po (1998: 52) defines the effectiveness of a drug as the 'extent to which it achieves its intended purpose for the broad range of patients who will receive it in practice'. This definition can be broadened to include consideration of treatments, procedures, therapies and services.

Health service policy-makers are putting more and more emphasis on the importance of using the latest and highest quality scientific evidence to inform the identification of clinical effectiveness. This is in fact one of the principle aims of UK NHS research and development policy (DoH 1996). Quite simply there is an enormous need for evidence about clinical effectiveness so that practitioners can choose appropriate treatments, managers are informed when making decisions about new services or modifying existing ones, and everyone can improve health outcomes for both individuals and the population as a whole. In a wider context of soaring health service costs due to both increasing demand and expensive technical advances there is also an increasing emphasis on issues of cost-effectiveness. The cost-effectiveness of a particular treatment is defined as the ratio of an intervention of proven effectiveness to its cost (NHSE 1996b; Muir Gray 1997). UK NHS policy suggests that: 'Only by choosing more cost effective services are we able to secure the greatest possible health gain for the resources available' (NHSE 1996b: 45).

Finding evidence

The thousands of medical and health care publications published throughout the world provide the raw information for the assessment of clinical and cost effectiveness. Much of this information uses the approaches, research designs and methods described in earlier chapters. It is estimated that there are currently 20,000 medical journals (Muir Gray 1997) and some believe that this number is growing exponentially. Considerable amounts of information are now also being disseminated in new ways given rapid developments in information technology. The World Wide Web and multimedia compact discs (CD-ROMs) are examples of new media that are gaining fast and widening use. Everyone is facing the problem of how to deal with ever-increasing volumes of information, and this problem is no less acute within the health care professions.

Journal indexes such as *Index Medicus* and *Excerpta Medica* provide regular listings of research articles published in scientific medical journals. *Index*

Medicus can be searched electronically using Medline (the National Library of Medicine's bibliographical databases), and **MeSH terms** – Medical Subject Headings – a thesaurus of nearly 18,000 main subjects that are used to classify articles and can be used to search for papers on a particular topic. Other examples of computer-based databases of health-related articles include:

- EMBASE, Elsevier Science's database of biomedicine
- CINAHL, Cumulative Index to Nursing and Allied Health Literature
- HealthSTAR, a database of literature about health services, technologies, administration and research
- SSCI and SCI, the Social Science and Science Citation Indexes, which allow users to track an article and see who else has cited it.

It should be noted that journal indexes and databases do not have complete blanket coverage. *Index Medicus*, Medline and Embase catalogue approximately 13.5 per cent, 18.5 per cent and 17.5 per cent of medical journals respectively. They focus mainly on journal articles written in English, although Embase has good European coverage (Muir Gray 1997). For these reasons it is sensible to use more than one database when carrying out literature searches.

A librarian's help is invaluable when undertaking exhaustive and specific searching. Librarians may provide guidance on the choice of appropriate MeSH terms for literature searches and also help modify and widen or narrow searches that do not yield good results. The main things to consider when undertaking a literature search are the search/MeSH terms and the search period (recent or going back a number of years). Box 8.1 provides

---

Box 8.1 Example of a Medline search

```
#1   explode 'AIR-POLLUTANTS, -ENVIRONMENTAL'/ all subheadings
#2   explode 'ASTHMA/ all subheadings
#3   REVIEW-ACADEMIC in PT
#4   REVIEW-TUTORIAL in PT
#5   META-ANALYSIS in PT
#6   'META-ANALYSIS'
#7   (SYSTEMATIC* near REVIEW*) in TI
#8   (SYSTEMATIC* near REVIEW*) in AB
#9   (SYSTEMATIC* near OVERREVIEW*) in TI
#10  (SYSTEMATIC* near OVERREVIEW*) in AB
#11  META? ANALY* in TI
#12  META? ANALY* in AB
#13  #3 or #4 or #5 or #6 or #7 or #8 or #9 or #10 or #11 or #12
#14  (TG=ANIMAL) not (TG=HUMAN)
#15  #13 not #14
#16  #1 and #2 and #15
```

Source: Muir Gray 1997.

an example of a Medline search strategy for finding systematic reviews on air pollutants and asthma.

The **Cochrane Library** is another computerized database that can be searched for systematic reviews, clinical trials and other EBHC information. It is made up of four databases (see Box 8.2) and can be found in most libraries and many hospital wards and departments. *Best Evidence* is a CD-ROM database that contains electronic copies of all articles published in *Evidence-based Medicine* and *American College of Physicians Journal Club.* The *National Research Register* is produced jointly by the NHS Executive R&D Directorate and the Medical Research Council, and contains information about ongoing and recently completed research projects.

Box 8.2   The Cochrane Library

- *Cochrane Database of Systematic Reviews (CDSR)*: a rapidly growing collection of updated systematic reviews (300 to date) prepared by contributors to the *Cochrane Collaboration.*
- *The York Database of Abstracts of Reviews of Effectiveness (DARE)*: this is an additional collection of over 100 abstracts of reviews from around the world which have been quality checked by the NHS Centre for Reviews and Dissemination (University of York).
- *Cochrane Controlled Trials Register (CCTR)*: a bibliography of over 100,000 randomized clinical trials.
- *Cochrane Review Methodology Database (CRMD)*: this contains a bibliography of articles on how to carry out systematic reviews.

Types of evidence

The quality and the strength of scientific evidence are dependent on the *research design* (see Chapters 3, 4 and 5). The best research designs reduce the susceptibility of a research study and its results to bias. Randomized clinical trials (RCTs) are considered to provide a 'gold standard' for answering questions about clinical effectiveness. RCTs (Chapter 4) involve the collection and comparison of clinical outcomes for both new experimental clinical 'interventions' and more traditional practices and control treatments (placebos and sham treatments) (Pocock 1983). In fact they can also be used to study care regimes, drug therapies, and surgical procedures. RCTs of the 'double blind' variety where neither the researcher nor patients/subjects know which treatments have been assigned to the latter are considered to provide the best evidence about efficacy. Biased results will be minimized if randomization is carried out appropriately and, if a large enough number of patients or subjects is recruited, the possibility of chance findings will be reduced (D'Agostino and Kwan 1995).

Other examples of research designs are more appropriate for answering other types of research question (Crombie and Davies 1996) or where it is neither possible nor practical to undertake a RCT. Longitudinal cohort studies provide reasonably strong evidence in the absence of RCTs when the time of exposure to a treatment or drug is known (i.e. other explanations for results will be less likely, although possible) and also because the patients are known to be drawn from the same population. Harrison *et al.* (1994) studied the long-term service needs and outcome of schizophrenics using a retrospective cohort of patients first seen between 1978 and 1980 (identified from medical records) and then subsequently traced and interviewed to determine their current heath status. Quite clearly an RCT would be inappropriate for long-term mental health outcomes (in this case over an average of 13 years).

Case-control studies are frequently used in epidemiology to answer questions about disease causation particularly where a condition is rare and the potential number of cases to be studied is small. Gardner *et al.*'s (1990b) methodological discussion of their case-control study of leukaemia and lymphoma among young people living near the Sellafield nuclear plant provides an excellent example (see Chapter 7). Cross-sectional studies provide the best ways of finding out about the accuracy of a diagnostic test (Sackett *et al.* 1997). Results for patients using a 'new' diagnostic test are compared (where possible blindly) with those obtained using the current conventional 'reference' test (Box 8.3). Qualitative study designs are very useful for providing 'thick' (detailed, contextualized) descriptions and explanations for people's motivations and reasons for their actions in particular situations and contexts (Sayer 1992). For example, the accounts provided by qualitative studies will provide richer insights and explanations for why the modification or introduction of a new service fails to deliver anticipated benefits.

Table 8.1 provides a summary and classification of 'best evidence'. So far we have only considered the nature and design of individual studies as published sources of evidence about clinical effectiveness (Types II–IV). We consider systematic reviews, which synthesize the results and findings of a number of different studies (Type I), in a later section. Whilst it has been argued that published evidence from well designed research studies is very important for health care decision making, that is not to say that clinical experience and scientific reasoning do not have important roles. An example is provided by a Brazilian doctor who saved a patient who was bleeding to death three weeks after bypass surgery by using 'superglue' imaginatively (*The Times* 16 March 1998). Usual techniques including sutures and surgical glue for holding surgical patches in place had failed, but the doctor 'recalled how his seven-year-old son had glued his fingers together when playing with "Super Bonder" a household glue'. The doctor would not recommend future use and said: 'I did something which had no scientific basis out of sheer desperation'.

It should be noted that there is an ever-increasing number of newsletters, briefings and websites (for example, *Evidence-based Nursing, Evidence-based Medicine, Clinical Evidence, American College of Physicians Journal Club, Bandolier, Evidence Matters, Evidence-based Purchasing* and *Outcomes Briefing*) that provide summarized EBHC information. They typically summarize

---

Box 8.3 Some measures of effectiveness in screening studies

	True status	
Classified by test as:	*With disease*	*Without disease*
Having disease	155	29
Not having disease	52	165

True positives = 155   False positives = 29
False negatives = 52   True negatives = 165

Sensitivity: the percentage of persons with the disease of interest who have positive test results.

$$\text{Sensitivity} = \frac{155}{155 + 52} = 0.75 \text{ (or 75\%)}$$

Specificity: the percentage of persons without the disease of interest who have negative test results.

$$\text{Specificity} = \frac{165}{165 + 29} = 0.85 \text{ (or 85\%)}$$

A sensitive test has relatively few false negatives, and a specific test relatively few false positives. The greater the sensitivity of a test, the more likely that the test will detect persons with the disease of interest.

Likelihood ratio (LR): a measure of how much more *likely* a person is to have a disease if they have had a positive test result.

$$\text{Likelihood ratio} = \frac{\text{Sensitivity}}{1.0 - \text{Specificity}} = 5$$

How many 'times more likely' a person with a positive test is to have the disease than someone who tests negative. As a guide LR > 10 or LR < 0.1 are useful in either justifying a test or rejecting it.

Positive predictive value (PV$^+$): the probability of persons with positive test results actually having the disease of interest

$$PV^+ = \frac{155}{155 + 29} = 0.84 \text{ (or 84\%)}$$

Negative predictive value (PV$^-$): the probability of persons with negative test results not actually having the disease.

$$PV^- = \frac{165}{165 + 52} = 0.76 \text{ (or 76\%)}$$

Table 8.1 Strength of evidence

Type	Strength of evidence
I	Strong evidence from at least one systematic review of multiple well designed randomized controlled trials
II	Strong evidence from at least one well designed randomized controlled trial of appropriate size
III	Evidence from well designed trials without randomization (follow-up, cohort/longitudinal, or matched case-control studies)
IV	Evidence from well designed non-experimental studies from more than one centre or research group
V	Opinions of respected authorities, based on clinical experience, descriptive studies or reports of experts committees

Source: Muir Gray 1997.

key results from a single study or a systematic review of several trials, as well as some methodological articles. They are invaluable resources for busy health care professions given the rapid increase in the number of journal publications.

Systematic reviews

The strongest evidence about clinical effectiveness (Type I in Table 8.1) is provided when different research studies are combined in a **systematic review** of all relevant previous research studies on a particular topic (Muir Gray 1997). Results from a single research study provide limited evidence about clinical effectiveness for a number of reasons. First, when studies are based on a small sample of patients (observations, or clinics, etc.) results may be imprecise and the findings may be due to chance. Secondly, whilst a single large drug trial may demonstrate that a particular treatment or therapy is efficacious, the conditions in which it is carried out might be somewhat artificial and not representative of what would be achieved if the new treatment were carried out in other everyday settings. Finally, a single research study can often be limited in scope and not provide the full picture necessary to make a fully informed decision about a particular health intervention. For example, when considering the efficacy of nicotine replacement therapy for preventing smoking it is important to base decisions on information drawn from all relevant studies that have considered possible interventions.

Good reviews will involve some investigation and description of the similarities and discrepancies in results between different studies. Moreover, they will statistically combine results, to facilitate an improvement in the accuracy of estimates of clinical effectiveness. For a review to be useful and reliable, it also needs to be carried out rigorously and with attention to publication bias – where the nature, direction, and statistical significance of results influences decisions about the submission and publication of research findings. These issues can be addressed by searching for all studies using systematic and comprehensive literature searches (see above). Sackett *et al.* (1991) are critical of many reviews, suggesting that the reasons for their deficiencies: 'lie in the tradition of calling upon content-area experts to produce them . . . these authors begin their task with a conclusion . . . and there is little wonder then that the results may be skewed'.

The International Cochrane Collaboration and the NHS CRD (Centre for Reviews and Dissemination) produces high quality systematic reviews that follow internationally accepted guidelines (CRD 1996; Chalmers and Altman 1995). The key features of such reviews are:

- the methodology used is fully described in a protocol, so that the review is reproducible and can be updated in the future;
- the materials used are obtained from systematic and exhaustive searches of published and unpublished studies, including sources written in foreign languages;
- the rationale and criteria for inclusion and exclusion are clearly defined;
- studies included in the review are systematically appraised (see below) and the methods used are made explicit. Where possible, objective scoring systems are used to assess methodological quality (for example, Chalmers *et al.* 1985; Mile and Chambers 1993);
- the analysis of results is based on appropriate techniques that are well documented;
- **meta-analysis** is commonly used to combine and analyse results (see next section);
- there is a commentary on the clinical significance of the results;
- the results of the systematic review are peer reviewed.

Meta-analysis

Meta-analysis is a statistical technique used to assemble results from several studies and create a single estimate for a particular health outcome (for example, stopping smoking). Results from different studies are pooled so that more weight is given to data derived from larger studies (where chance findings are less likely). The overall estimate of clinical effectiveness (based on all studies) is typically an odds ratio, and is presented together with a confidence interval – the range of values in which the true value will lie.

Meta-analysis results are best presented graphically as in Figure 8.1, where four outcome measures for sustained abstinence from smoking and point prevalence of non-smoking at 6 and 12 months are shown for several trials of nicotine patches. Estimates of clinical efficacy (the dark notches) are shown study by study using odds ratios, together with their confidence intervals (whiskers); and the overall subtotals and totals are illustrated by rectangles and diamonds, with their widths portraying confidence intervals. Notice that only the studies by Hurt make use of all four outcome measures. The vertical line that passes through the diagram represents an odds ratio of 1, where the treatment effect is the same in the

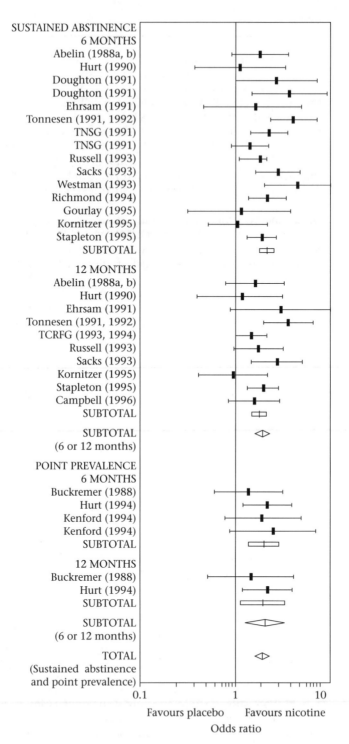

Figure 8.1 Meta-analysis of odds ratios and associated 95 per cent confidence for the effect of nicotine patch on smoking cessation.
Source: Li Wan Po 1998.

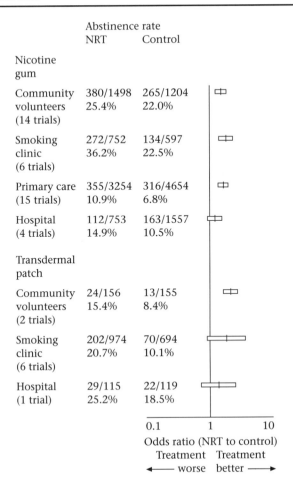

Abstinence rate
NRT   Control

Nicotine
gum

Community   380/1498 265/1204
volunteers 25.4%   22.0%
(14 trials)

Smoking   272/752   134/597
clinic   36.2%   22.5%
(6 trials)

Primary care 355/3254 316/4654
(15 trials) 10.9%   6.8%

Hospital   112/753   163/1557
(4 trials) 14.9%   10.5%

Transdermal
patch

Community   24/156   13/155
volunteers 15.4%   8.4%
(2 trials)

Smoking   202/974   70/694
clinic   20.7%   10.1%
(6 trials)

Hospital   29/115   22/119
(1 trial)   25.2%   18.5%

0.1   1   10
Odds ratio (NRT to control)
Treatment   Treatment
◄— worse   better —►

Figure 8.2 Efficacy of nicotine gum and transdermal patches in different
clinical settings. (Odds ratios are shown by vertical lines and 95 per cent
confidence intervals by width of boxes.)
Source: Silagy *et al.* 1994.

intervention and control groups. Odds ratios to the right of the line
represent results where the clinical effect is greater in the intervention group
than the treatment group, there being more abstinence or prevalence of
non-smoking, and suggest that nicotine replacement therapy is effective.
Odds ratios to left of the line represent the reverse situation of less abstinence or prevalence of non-smoking and favour the placebo. If the outcome
measure was prevalence of smoking, an odds ratio to the left of the line
would favour the use of nicotine patches. Confidence intervals which have
long whiskers represent studies that are based on a small number of patients
and have imprecise results; and those that cut the line of no treatment
effect are not statistically significant (for example, Gourlay's study).
    Figure 8.2 shows the results of the efficacy of nicotine gum and
transdermal patches in different clinical settings and it is only possible to

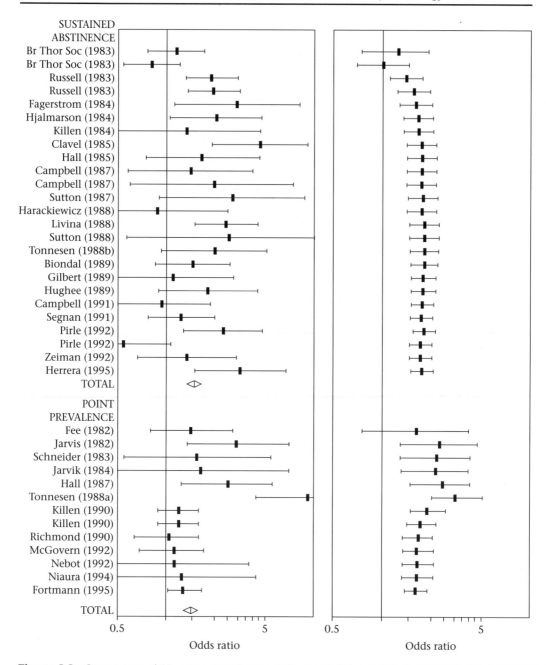

Figure 8.3 Comparison of (a) conventional meta-analysis and (b) cumulative meta-analysis of nicotine chewing gum on smoking cessation at 12 months.
Source: Li Wan Po 1998.

compare results between different types of trial. This less detailed display is typical of those used for the meta-analyses published in the Cochrane Library. The logo for the International Cochrane Collaboration is a meta-analysis diagram contained within a circle representing the globe.

Figure 8.3 provides a comparison of a conventional meta-analysis with a cumulative Mantel–Haenszel meta-analysis, where studies are presented sequentially. The diagram shows that after completion of the first three trials, a statistically significant pooled estimate of nicotine chewing gum efficacy could have been obtained. As more studies are combined there is an increase in precision of the pooled estimate. Antman et al. (1992) provide another example that shows the results of 17 RCTs of the effects of oral beta-blockers on secondary prevention of mortality amongst patients who have survived myocardial infarction (heart attack). The traditional diagram shows several non-significant results, whilst the cumulative diagram shows a statistically significant pooled estimate in 1977 after four trials (involving a total of 5322 patients). It is interesting to note that such thrombolytic therapy was not routinely recommended in medical textbooks until the mid-1980s. This retrospective analysis provides a classical example of the inherent time-lag in getting new evidence into practice.

Appraising published research evidence

It is not always easy to make quick judgements about research findings published in journal articles and systematic reviews. We need to ask whether published studies contain strong evidence to suggest changing practice in local health care settings. Some specific questions about research articles arise:

- Was the research design used appropriate?
- Was the methodology vigorous?
- Was the analysis presented valid?
- What is the applicability of the results to a local setting?

Several sets of structured questions and guidelines for reviewing health-based research are now available (Guyatt and Rennie 1993; Greenhalgh and Taylor 1997; Muir Gray 1997; Sackett et al. 1997). Box 8.4 summarizes three such schemata; we have already covered a further approach in Chapter 7, that of Elwood (1998). Dixon et al. (1997) provide an alternative set of questions for critically appraising clinical literature in a problem-centred workbook. Greenhalgh (1997) provides more general tips and guidance on critical reading in what is a particularly easy to read account. Structured questions are also available for assessing cohort studies, diagnostic/screening tests, decision analysis, cost effectiveness/economic evaluation, and health care polices (see Muir Gray 1997).

Box 8.5 provides an example of the application of the ten questions for assessing systematic reviews to Silagy et al.'s (1994) review of the efficacy of nicotine replacement therapy (NRT). The review is vigorous and trustworthy and suggests that NRT is effective in helping people give up smoking. Number needed to treat (NNT) is a measure of clinical effectiveness

Box 8.4   Structured approaches to appraising research articles

A. *Ten questions to help you make sense of a single research study*
  1 Did the article address a clearly focused issue?
  2 Was the study designed in a way which allowed it to address the issue?
  3 Was patient selection carried out appropriately?
  4 Was the study designed appropriately?
  5 Was the study conducted and analysed appropriately?
  6 What are the results of the study?
  7 How precise are the results?
  8 Can the results be applied to your patients?
  9 Were all important outcomes considered?
10 Are the benefits worth the harms and costs?

B. *Ten questions to help you make sense of a systematic review*
  1 Did the review address a clearly focused issue?
  2 Did the authors select the right sorts of study for the review?
  3 Do you think the important, relevant studies were included?
  4 Did the review's authors do enough to assess the quality of the included studies?
  5 If the results of the review have been combined, was it reasonable to do so?
  6 What is the overall result of the review?
  7 How precise are the results?
  8 Can the results be applied to the local population?
  9 Were all important outcomes considered?
10 Are the benefits worth the harms and costs?

C. *Nine questions to help evaluate papers that describe qualitative research*
  1 Did the paper describe an important clinical problem addressed via a clearly formulated question?
  2 Was a qualitative approach appropriate?
  3 How were the setting and the subjects selected?
  4 What was the researcher's perspective, and has this been taken into account?
  5 What methods did the researcher use for collecting data, and are these described in enough detail?
  6 What methods did the researcher use to analyse the data, and what quality control measures were implemented?
  7 Are the results credible, and if so, are they clinically important?
  8 What conclusions were drawn, and are they justified by the results?
  9 Are the findings of the study transferable to other clinical settings?

Source: A, Guyatt *et al.* 1993, 1994; B, based on Oxman *et al.* 1994; C, Greenhalgh and Taylor 1997.

Box 8.5 A summary critical appraisal of Silagy *et al.*'s (1994) review of the efficacy of nicotine replacement therapy

1 *Did the review address a clearly focused issue?*
The question tackled was 'how effective is NRT?' and was stated at the beginning of the abstract and again at the end of the introduction. The population studied was people who wanted to give up smoking in a variety of clinical settings. A number of different forms of NRT were studied (chewing gum, patches, sprays and inhalers). The outcome measures studied were proportion quitting and abstinence rates (with biochemical confirmation where possible). Side-effects were not considered.

2 *Did the authors select the right sorts of study for the review?*
Studies included were appropriate and had at least one treatment group and a control group, with random or quasi-random allocation. Studies that made use of historical controls were excluded.

3 *Do you think the important, relevant studies were included?*
The search strategy was comprehensive and included: seven databases; reference lists from clinical trials; conference abstracts; smoking-and-health bulletins; and a bibliography. The authors also wrote to drug manufacturers asking about unpublished data.

4 *Did the review's authors do enough to assess the quality of the included studies?*
The methodological quality of the studies was assessed using Chalmer's criteria (Chalmers *et al.* 1985). The authors noted that the extent to which bias was controlled varied between trials, and that randomization was not described in 39 of the trials studied. Similarly, only 12 of the studies involved blinded validation of smoking status and only 21 studies reported smoking status at final follow-up. People who were lost to follow-up were defined as continuing smokers.

5 *Were the results similar from study to study?*
The results were very consistent, despite variations in study design, clinical setting, dosage regime, outcome measurement and losses to follow-up. There was no statistically significant variation in results between studies.

6 *What is the overall result of the review?*
The quantitative meta-analysis undertaken suggested that NRT is an effective intervention (overall odds ratio = 1.71). Effects were greatest for nicotine inhalers, followed by sprays, patches and gum, and highest for those with higher dependency (although not significantly). Treatments were effective in all the settings quoted. Numbers needed to treat (NNT) were also reported for different forms of NRT, clinical setting and intensity of support.

7 *How precise are the results?*
The overall result is based on data for 18,000 subjects and is therefore precise with a small confidence interval (1.56 to 1.87). Confidence intervals for odds ratios associated with inhaler and spray are larger as there was only one reported trial in each case. Estimates of numbers needed to treat with NRT are also reported in a table, together with confidence intervals.

8 *Can the results be applied to the local population?*
The review suggests that NRT is effective in a wide range of clinical settings. There is some discussion of whether nicotine patches are superior to gum, but results are neither conclusive nor statistically significant. Benefits do seem to be greater for those with higher dependency and those motivated to quit (for example, community volunteers and patients attending smoking cessation clinics). There is no reason to think that the patients studied would be different from those treated in local settings.

9 *Were all clinically important outcomes considered? If not, does this affect the decision?*
The main outcome considered was quitting smoking. The side-effects of treatment were not considered.

10 *Are the benefits worth the harms and costs?*
This was not considered and there was no information on costs.

which complements the odds ratio, but can be interpreted more easily by health practitioners. It is the number of people you would need to treat with a specific intervention (for example, nicotine gum for smokers) to see a single occurrence of a specific outcome (for example, stopping smoking). The calculation of NNT is described in Box 8.6 and can also be used to estimate the risk of harm. Based on data contained in Silagy *et al.* (1994), it is estimated that if at least one patient is to stop smoking then approximately 13 smokers would need to be treated with nicotine gum.

Conclusion

This chapter has considered sources of evidence, searching for evidence, and critically reviewing and appraising evidence. At the beginning of this chapter it was noted that interest in EBHC was clinically focused and concerned with the best ways of treating and managing individual patients. Grol (1997) describes 'epidemiological approaches' to changing practice as involving summarizing sound scientific literature and developing vigorous and valid clinical guidelines. The interface between EBHC and epidemiology and public health medicine should be obvious, but is reinforced by the government's recognition that there is a need for: 'Refocusing research

---

Box 8.6 Calculating number needed to treat

Calculating NNT
1 Calculate the proportion of people who have the outcome in the *new intervention* group, that is the experimental group event rate (EER).
2 Calculate the proportion of people who have the outcome in the *placebo* or *control* group, that is the control group event rate (CER).
3 Calculate the difference between the CER and EER to determine the absolute risk reduction (ARR). This gives you the percentage of people helped by the treatment.
4 To find the numbers needed to treat, take the reciprocal of the ARR:

$$NNT = \frac{1}{ARR}$$

Worked example
Silagy *et al.* (1994: table 1) report that 1456 out of 7834 smokers who were given nicotine replacement therapy stopped smoking in randomized controlled trials compared with 1016 out of 9600 smokers given placebos.

1 EER $= \dfrac{1456}{7834} = 0.1858$

2 CER $= \dfrac{1916}{9600} = 0.1058$

3 AAR $=$ EER $-$ CER $= 0.1858 - 0.1058 = 0.08$

4 NNT $= \dfrac{1}{ARR} = \dfrac{1}{0.08} = 12.5 \approx 13$

---

and development on public health issues, rather than just health care' (DoH 1998b: 42). The skills, methods, techniques and information resources (such as systematic reviews) described in this chapter are central to facilitating and practising evidence-based health care and getting research findings into practice (Glanville *et al.* 1998; Staus and Sackett 1998).

Summary

- Epidemiological evidence is central to evidence-based health care and provides the basic techniques applied in the practice of evidence-based health care.

- The thousands of medical and health care publications published throughout the world provide the raw information for the assessment of clinical and cost effectiveness. Journal indexes such as *Index Medicus/*

Medline and *Excerpta Medica*/Embase provide frequently published listings of research articles published in scientific medical journals. The Cochrane Library can be searched for systematic reviews, clinical trials and other evidence-based health care information.

● The best research designs reduce the susceptibility of a research study and its results to bias. Randomized clinical trials (RCTs) are considered to provide a 'gold standard' for answering questions about clinical effectiveness. Results from a single research study provide limited evidence about clinical effectiveness, however. Systematic reviews synthesize the results and findings of a number of different studies and usually focus on RCTs.

● Meta-analysis is a statistical technique used to assemble results from several studies and to create a single estimate for a particular health outcome (for example, stopping smoking).

● Several sets of structured questions and guidelines for reviewing health-based research are now available. Structured questions are also available for assessing cohort studies, diagnostic/screening tests, decision analysis, cost effectiveness/economic evaluation, and health care.

Further reading

Chalmers, I. and Altman, D. (eds) (1995) *Systematic Reviews*. London: BMJ Publishing Group.

Cochrane, A. (1972) *Effectiveness and Efficiency: Random Reflections on Health Services*. London: Nuffield Provincial Hospital Trust.

Muir Gray, J. (1997) *Evidence-based Healthcare: How to Make Health Policy and Management Decisions*. Edinburgh: Churchill Livingstone.

Sackett, D., Haynes, R. and Tugwell, P. (eds) (1991) *Clinical Epidemiology: A Basic Science For Clinical Medicine*, 2nd edition. Boston: Little Brown.

Sackett, D., Richardson, W., Rosenburg, W. and Haynes, R. (1997) *Evidence-based Medicine: How to Practice and Teach EBM*. Edinburgh: Churchill Livingstone.

Activities

1 In the activities for Chapter 2, we talked about the hypothesis that unhealthy diet may cause heart disease. Thinking now of your own professional interests, try to identify a similar causal hypothesis for a disease or health condition of your choice. Try to specify the search terms you might use to find different sorts of published studies on this topic, for example different sorts of epidemiological design. If you have access to the necessary resources, try out your search strategy using Medline or a similar bibliographical database. Note that you will need to become familiar with using the database first. Note too that you may

find thousands of references – or none. If such extreme outcomes happen, you will need to think about how you might change your search strategy.

2 Looking back over the past chapters, comment critically on the notion of a hierarchy of scientific evidence. What do you think it says about the concerns of evidence-based health care? Does it have any negative consequences?

3 Try to get hold of a copy of systematic review relevant to your professional interests. Does it raise any implications for your current practice? If it does, discuss these implications with your work colleagues.

4 Calculate the NNT for the data below.

	Treated	Not treated	Total
Cured	91	23	114
Not cured	287	325	612
Total	378	348	726

NINE

BRINGING IN CONTEXT AND PEOPLE

The study of health and illness is a subject that requires multiple perspectives and multiple approaches. In this chapter we move back from the formal, and some might say medicalized, concern with critical appraisal and the assessment of epidemiological evidence with which we were concerned in the previous chapter, and re-engage with the more critical position on epidemiological evidence which we introduced in Chapter 7. More specifically, we are concerned to show that different questions, 'accounts', and 'ways of knowing' can be applied to epidemiological problems. In addressing this focus we draw upon a much more sociological literature than that cited in previous chapters.

The chapter explores both *critical* and *lay* (or popular) approaches to epidemiology. Following a short consideration of a range of arguments, largely emanating from within the discipline itself, which have called into question some of the underlying principles upon which modern epidemiology is based, we will consider critical epidemiology. The particular focus of attention will be on epidemiology's failure to take account of its 'positivistic' theoretical stance. This failure, we will argue, has left epidemiology ill-equipped to explain the role of wider social processes in the patterning of health and illness. Following this we look at lay epidemiology. We will consider how the general public interprets and reconstructs traditional epidemiological 'facts' in order to make them more useful to their own understanding of health risks, illness and disease within their own particular social contexts.

By the end of the chapter you should be able to:

- define and appreciate the epistemological context of modern epidemiology;
- appreciate the case for a critical epidemiology;
- recognize the importance of lay epidemiology.

The epistemological context of modern epidemiology

Within western society it could be argued that a biomedical perspective dominates within the field of epidemiology. Epidemiology is thought of as the 'science of epidemics' or, more explicitly, the study of disease and illness and risk factors as they occur in populations (Peterson and Lupton 1996). It is portrayed as a 'neutral science' based upon measurement and quantification. Fundamental critiques of epidemiology as science have emanated from individuals such as Treichler (1988, 1992), Lupton (1995, 1997) and Petersen and Lupton (1996). Presuming these critiques to be accurate (and in many respects they are often unjust and partial), a number of problems arise.

First, few would dispute that the real foundations of epidemiology were laid in the nineteenth century. The subject matter for its classic studies was outbreaks of infectious/communicable diseases like cholera and tuberculosis. These diseases laid low vast sections of the population of Britain and recurred in cycles – or epidemics. In this sense, epidemiology was indeed originally the study of epidemics of infectious disease. As epidemiology has moved away from these *public health* origins, it has increasingly become focused upon the explanatory power of its methods rather than upon the people it studies. Popay and Williams (1996) and Armstrong (1993) suggest that epidemiology has forgotten its initial commitments to social improvement in its increasing stress upon methodology. An editorial of *The Lancet* (Anon. 1994), suggested that the discipline's focus is now so far 'downstream' that it has lost sight of what is going on up river. The result is an exclusion of the *contexts* in which disease happens unless they are immediately measurable, and the *voices* of those people whose social conditions threaten their health, placing them at risk of illness and disease.

Secondly, central to current epidemiology is the notion of 'population surveillance' (Foucault 1984: 278). This is directed at identifying patterns of disease at the population level in order to find out why certain groups develop particular conditions. In other words, epidemiology attempts to assess the health of a community. Using a web of causation, epidemiology draws data from many different sources (for example, medical records, cross-sectional surveys, cohort studies, case comparison studies and clinical trials) in order to create statistical records of a particular health problem. In so doing, epidemiology makes these problems calculable, or 'real', and subsequently subject to diagnosis and intervention (Rose and Miller 1992). Unfortunately, however, the result is a tendency to make people and their sociocultural contexts 'disappear'. While epidemiology is a powerful tool for exploring patterns of illness and disease, it ignores people and the social contexts in which they live, and becomes seriously limited in its ability to bring about changes in these patterns.

A common theme found within much of the discussion surrounding the nature of modern epidemiology is its close relationship with biomedical science. At one level this should not appear as problematic given that epidemiology might be considered to be the 'basic science of public health' (Wing 1994) and, as such, is responsible for explaining the occurrence of disease in populations. However, as contemporary epidemiology has

Table 9.1 Epidemiological paradigms

	Traditional epidemiology	Modern epidemiology
Motivation	Public health	Science
Level of study	Population	Individuals/organ/tissue/cell/molecule
Context of study	Historical/cultural	(Often) Context free
Designs and disciplines	Cross-sectional: demography/social science	Medical science: experimental studies
Epistemological strategy	Top-down (structural)	Bottom-up (reductionist)
Level of intervention	Population (upstream)	Individual (downstream)

Source: adapted from Pearce 1996.

broken away from its traditional links with public health, its practitioners have given greater value to the explanatory power of their methodological tools than to the people, the populations, they ultimately seek to serve (Pearce 1996; Frankenberg 1994; Lupton 1995). The result(s) of this shift in paradigm are presented in Table 9.1.

In Table 9.1 the **epistemological strategy** of modern epidemiology (the way in which the discipline constructs knowledge) is shown to impact upon the discipline's explanatory power in a number of important ways. First, the level of study is shown to have shifted from the population to the individual; a movement which might be seen to have gone even further given the emergence of 'molecular' and 'genetic' epidemiology (Loomis and Wing 1991; Diez-Roux 1998). This removes the individual from the context in which his or her health is experienced. It is related to the problem of aggregating data collected on individuals into groups unsuitable for causal analysis. An example might be the use of such 'natural' descriptors as 'homosexual/bisexual', 'intravenous drug user', 'heterosexual', 'Black African' and 'Haitian' in the creation of bounded population sub-groups 'at risk' from HIV/AIDS (Schiller *et al.* 1994). Another example is that of social class whereby individuals are grouped by their occupation and other supposedly shared attributes. Such group markers are largely constructed for ease of analysis. The individuals in the groups might only have one attribute or 'risk factor' in common: their sexuality, their ethnicity, their drug use, their occupation or whatever. Such ordering of a (dis)orderly social world is seen as inherently problematic (Lupton 1995).

Another point raised by Table 9.1 is that epidemiology has adopted the **reductionist principles** upon which modern science is based, an approach whereby the factors of disease are viewed in isolation from their context, and complex interactions are reduced to component parts. The key point here is that, within a medical context, reductionism contributes to a belief that the true cause of illness is to be found inside the biological body – in the biological mechanisms that cause disease – and that the 'true' causes of disease are exclusively within individuals (Diez-Roux 1998). The postulates of causality set out in Chapter 4 very explicitly contribute to this point in their call for biological plausibility. In this way, individuals as dehumanized subjects are removed from their physical and social environments and reduced to the 'risk factors' identified in epidemiological explanations. Brown (1995) suggests that human populations become mere 'dots on maps'; their contexts are obscured and their voices ignored. If a more robust and holistic explanation for such patterns in society is to emerge, research in this area must incorporate both sociocultural context and people's lay knowledge and understanding of health risk, illness and disease.

Critical epidemiology

Critical epidemiology might be argued to have emerged first in the 1980s when a series of articles were published in the journal then titled *Radical Community Medicine* (now *Critical Public Health*). Emerging from a concern over the biomedical focus of modern or 'orthodox' epidemiology, the arguments for a 'critical' approach have remained largely within the bounds of epidemiology as the 'study of disease in relation to populations' (Rose and Barker 1986). That is to say, the proponents of a critical epidemiology seek to distance the discipline from some of the key problems associated with positivistic biomedical science but not to divorce it from such an approach entirely. In this sense, concern is neither with the scientific construction of 'facts' nor with the scientific 'ordering' of the social world. Rather, a critical epidemiology seeks to move towards an approach which takes account of the 'social structures and processes within which ill health originates' (Jones and Moon 1987; Anon. 1994).

Such a response to orthodox epidemiology represents both a step forward and a leap backwards. The emphasis on societal structure reflects the concerns of mid-to-late nineteenth century public health medicine as it was championed by individuals such as Chadwick, Snow and, more relevantly, by Engels and Virchow. Following Pearce (1996), we might suggest that this early epidemiology was a branch of public health that was focused more directly on the causes and prevention of disease in populations whereas the focus in modern orthodox epidemiology is on individuals in abstraction from their social, economic, cultural, historical or political context. The reasons for this desire to return to a more socially activist epidemiology are not, however, purely ideological despite early calls for a 'socialist' epidemiology (Scott-Samuel 1981), a 'materialist' epidemiology (Jones and Moon 1987) or, more recently, for public health as a whole to embrace the challenges of a new social justice (Krieger and Birn 1998). Rather, they reflect a dual belief that epidemiology in its current form not only upholds the values of the dominant system within which it is practised but also that it is based upon flawed methodological assumptions associated with positivistic science.

Moreover, calls for a critical epidemiology also represent a view that epidemiological science has not necessarily achieved the aims that it has set for itself. Further, as an editorial in *The Lancet* states, research in epidemiology is dominated by a concern with experimental and quasi-experimental research designs that are based on simplistic notions of causality which seek to remove the variation and complexity of real-life health and disease processes (Anon. 1994). On the one hand, such models have been successful in producing clear links between individual risk factors and disease. One such example would be the case-control and cohort studies conducted by Sir Richard Doll and his colleagues on smoking and lung cancer (Doll and Hill 1954; Doll and Peto 1976, 1981). Yet, as Frankenberg (1994) argues, despite the power of such models, other more appealing rhetorics have meant that a large number of smokers remain in the UK and elsewhere.

This suggestion, that epidemiology has failed in its major task, is a point taken up by Syme (1996) who argues that even where epidemiological explanation is at its most successful, its conclusions are of relatively little significance. For example, in the case of risk factors for coronary heart disease (CHD), the discipline has succeeded in accounting for only 40 per cent of all CHD that occurs. While this represents a large number of people, it is still less than 50 per cent of disease prevalence. If we accept the view that modern epidemiology is increasingly focused on weak relationships and low-level exposures, of which passive smoking and environmental radiation are examples, the problems outlined by Syme become greatly magnified. The point here is that while individual-level factors are seen to be important, their explanatory power is limited because they tell us very little about the structural forces which impact upon the lives of a population. A useful example of this comes once again from epidemiology's successful account of the causal relationship between lung cancer and smoking tobacco.

According to Wing (1994), three distinct trends can be recognized in the global patterns of smoking prevalence and the occurrence of smoking-related diseases. The first is that among better educated, higher income groups in many western industrialized nations smoking prevalence has declined. This success is marred by the implications of a second trend that suggests that among the lower educated and lower income groups located within these very same countries the prevalence of smoking remains high. The third trend identified by Wing relates to the rapid increase in both smoking and smoking-related diseases, particularly in some of the most populous regions of the world. The key issue here is that by focusing on individual-level behaviours, of which cigarette smoking is just one, epidemiology has neglected the significant role played by the tobacco agribusiness, the commercial sales of cigarettes and the social circumstances that surround smoking. For Wing, the result of this focus on the consumption rather than the production and promotion of cigarettes has been a partial redistribution of smoking prevalence as tobacco companies redirect their commercial focus to newly expanding markets.

While it is still the case that critical epidemiology remains relatively underdeveloped, a growing body of work has been conducted which seeks to explain how such contextual issues impact upon individual-level risk behaviours. Such work recognizes not only the role(s) played by multinational companies in the production and consumption of health and illness, but also the importance of other social processes and forces which structure an individual's ability to make choices. It might be argued, following Krieger et al. (1993), that such choices are related to three underlying principles and assumptions. The first is associated with the belief in the social, and not the biological, production of divisions based on race, sex and class. As a consequence it is social factors, not genetics, that are seen to offer the primary explanation of why membership of these groups can help to predict overall health status. The second principle is that these social relations should be seen to have a direct impact on the health and illness of individuals on both sides of the divide, 'whites as well as blacks and other people of colour, men as well as women, and business owners and professionals as well as working-class employees' (Krieger *et al.* 1993). The final principle or assumption is that the mechanisms responsible are seen to exist at both the social and biological levels and, as a result, both levels must be studied in order to understand current and changing patterns of health and illness.

As we have already implied, there are problems associated with over-reliance on such broad categories, particularly the tendency to ignore the individual in favour of the structural. Keeping these problems in mind, we wish to draw upon two studies that explore the impact of structural forces upon our understanding of HIV/AIDS. The first is taken from Zierler and Krieger (1998), who argue that risk of AIDS among women in the USA is bound up with economic and social relations of power and control. Drawing on alternatives to biomedical, lifestyle and psychological models of disease causation, the authors suggest that inequalities are structured in relation to class, sex, race/ethnicity and sexuality and these affect an individual's risk of, and resistance to, HIV infection. In addition, Zierler and Krieger are particularly keen to stress the need to locate these inequalities in a framework which recognizes that such processes are played out at multiple spatial levels and during differing times of an individual's life course (Table 9.2).

The second example comes from the work of Paul Farmer (1992, 1996), whose emphasis remains on the structural but which, in contrast to Zierler and Krieger, involves the use of anthropological methods to gain a greater understanding of individual experience(s). Farmer asks: 'By what mechanisms do social forces ranging from poverty to racism become embodied as individual experience?' (Farmer 1996). In recounting the stories of two Haitian peasants, Farmer is not simply providing anecdotal evidence about the impact of HIV/AIDS on two individuals (both of whom died); rather, his account provides an insight into the role played by the one factor these individuals shared – abject poverty. This is an important issue, especially given that traditional epidemiology played a crucial role in the construction of Haiti as a 'risk group' for AIDS. Anthropological studies such as this bring into relief important relationships between exposure and disease (ill health) and broader structural forces. For Farmer, while each story is unique, there remains a 'deadly monotony' to them, a monotony which, for example, sees young women whose desire to escape the rural poverty they suffer drives them to Haiti's capital Port-au-Prince and prostitution. While this relationship is not necessarily causal it would appear difficult to argue that poverty does not play a part in the exposure of individuals to the HIV virus. Certainly, and this is the crucial point about such intensive qualitative studies, it provides for far greater understanding of the (human) dimensions of AIDS/HIV than more traditional epidemiological studies.

While it is important for a critical approach to avoid the 'romantic confusions and pseudo-Marxist mysticisms' which Frankenberg (1994) warns

Table 9.2　The impact of structural processes on women's experiences of HIV/AIDS

Structural process	Impact
Economic inequality	• Poverty and lack of resources keep individuals in areas of high HIV seroprevalence • Urban decay – crisis in housing, depleted budgets, poor schools, unemployment and other social problems – linked to high HIV prevalence
Racial inequality/racism	• Excess relative risk of AIDS among communities of colour reflect underlying discrimination in employment, housing, earning power, educational opportunity • Impact of prejudice on (mis)use of prescription and non-prescription drugs and possible association with HIV infection through sexual activity/intravenous drug use • Racism as a psychosocial stressor possibly linked with impairment of immune function
Sex inequalities	• Unequal sexual relations where the fear of loss of material support – food, housing, transportation – is associated with men who will not use condoms • Role of past or present violence in women's exposure to risk: 　– childhood sexual abuse and links to high risk sex, prostitution, use of crack, injection drug use, homelessness 　– fear of violence and links to women's inability to protect themselves sexually • Reduced autonomy in the social patterning of drug use. Women less likely to use needle exchange programmes because: 　– role of social norms on women's ability to obtain drugs and syringes 　– male partners preventing access 　– prevalence of street violence in areas where programmes located 　– problems of stigma associated with drug-using identity

Source: adapted from Zierler and Krieger 1998.

against, it is clear that the impact of structural forces on an individual's exposure to disease and ill health must be taken into account. This section of the chapter has given a number of examples of how we feel this might be achieved. However, this is not the only movement towards a reformed epidemiology that is currently taking place. Another movement, which has its roots in anthropological techniques, is lay epidemiology which involves community participation in the design and implementation of research and the development of subsequent interventions (Schwab and Syme 1997).

Lay epidemiology

By portraying itself as emerging from a neutral knowledge base supported by 'scientific methods', traditional epidemiology seeks to provide scientific objectivity, unstained by the entry of social or cultural values. Using the technical language of modern science, epidemiology constructs itself to be 'purely scientific' and therefore not influenced by sociocultural factors. However, what is often overlooked is that epidemiological research, like any other research, is a practice which involves 'constructing' problems, and defining and dealing with them in a specific way (Sayer 1992). The ways in which the problem is viewed shapes the 'facts' that ultimately emerge from the process or, as Jackson (1994) states, data gathered are data produced. Thus, facts are not autonomous entities but are constructed by human beings through knowledge and belief systems that are influenced by many different factors. For Fleck ([1936] 1979), facts are created collectively; they are a function of collective thinking varying through time and space. Consequently, it is necessary to recognize that epidemiological patterns are not simply 'out there' waiting to be uncovered by scientific methods. Rather, they are constructed through the expectations and processes of the people who study them. As Potter *et al.* (1991) suggest, decisions regarding whom to count, what to count and how to count it are made subjectively. In this sense, particular risk factors are identified as being 'problems' requiring measurement while others are ignored or downplayed.

This process of choosing which risk factors are important is itself affected by such sociocultural influences as current knowledge systems, the research interests of those involved and the interests of the funders of research. For example, it is generally assumed that there is a strong relationship between smoking and lung cancer and that smoking tobacco has no positive health properties. Research that seeks to demonstrate the positive effects of smoking tobacco is few and far between primarily because of a lack of available funding. Government funding bodies and researchers currently view tobacco as a 'bad' drug, and drug companies avoid funding research on a substance that is regarded by most people to be dangerous (Mundell 1993). Another example might be the pathologization of alcohol consumption as a health problem in North America. Alcohol consumption is usually portrayed as a negative and antisocial behaviour with no associated benefits despite epidemiological data which emphasize that the daily consumption of alcohol can reduce the risk of developing coronary heart disease (Peele 1993).

A further example of the socially constructed nature of epidemiological data is related to the ways in which the data are collected and analysed: as suggested earlier, epidemiological research creates categories into which people may be classified. The very act of classification also shapes the data collected. For example, when someone dies in the UK, a medical practitioner must complete a death certificate. It is, however, often the case that the cause(s) of death are imprecise or that death is due to a combination of social conditions rather than a single biomedical factor. In addition, changes in the rules for coding deaths can affect the production of mortality data; when sudden infant death syndrome was initially recognized as a category of death, the percentage of infant deaths attributed to other causes, such as pneumonia, fell. Thus, the accuracy of death certificate data is far from 'scientific' as it is based upon the judgement of individual medical practitioners (Prior and Bloor 1993).

This attempt by epidemiological research to 'slot' people within pre-established categories for the purpose of data collection also fails to recognize that individuals might resist classification and behave in ways that are outside of their given status. That is, they may not perceive themselves to be a particular social class despite their occupation, or they may hide or downplay behaviours such as unprotected sex or recreational drug-taking which are constructed as unhealthy or deviant. Consequently, epidemiological data are liable to 'contamination' often by the very subjects under surveillance.

Also contributing to the socially constructed character of traditional epidemiology is the underlying assumption that health, illness and disease are biological entities, static and unchanging, existing independently of sociocultural processes. Another account would see disease and illness as culturally constructed concepts interpreted through both lay and biomedical knowledge systems. This viewpoint does not seek to undermine the reality of illness and disease, or the linkages between them and associated variables such as age, sex, race and social class. Rather, it recognizes that the way in which such variables are measured, defined and represented as fact is subject to sociocultural processes. Such a recognition would not render disease or illness any less real or true but would enable their definition to be grounded 'in the lived experience of members of a shared culture' (Wright 1988: 299). Moreover, it would not privilege the biomedical account; rather, it would acknowledge that individual and collective popular/lay understandings are of equal merit – and often important in developing ways of treating or coping with disease.

The failure to take account of epidemiology's position within this power–knowledge nexus is best illustrated through an awareness of the continual renegotiation and revision that surrounds the clinical definition of health and illness. Some medical conditions, such as female hysteria, have been erased while others, such as passive smoking, have only recently appeared. In the case of the former, hysteria is seen to epitomize the cult of female invalidism. It affected middle and upper class women in nineteenth and early twentieth century Europe and North America, yet had no discernible organic basis and was totally resistant to medical treatment. While it could be argued that hysteria was related to the particular social and political environment of the time (Bassuk 1986), it might equally be argued that hysteria, like other representations of female madness, emerged as a consequence of the specific social relations of power from which the discipline of psychiatry emerged, and within which women were constructed as hysterical, irrational, or mad.

Passive smoking is a more recent example. Prior to the late 1970s little attention was given to the possible effects of passive smoking, with most attention being focused on the negative health impacts of tobacco on the individual smoker. However, by the late 1980s, and particularly by the 1990s, passive smoking was seen as a major health risk. As Jackson (1994) argues, biomedicine has constructed a scientific knowledge of tobacco smoke, a knowledge which, on the one hand, distinguishes between differing types of smoke and, on the other, classifies each type according to its individual chemical properties. In this way a scientific reality of tobacco smoke is created which enables epidemiology to establish causal links between passive smoking and known smoking-related illnesses. The point here is not to undermine the possibility that passive smoking is a potential risk to human health but rather to highlight the social, cultural and political processes that influence our understanding of health and illness.

As Beck (1996), Giddens (1991), Douglas and Wildavsky (1982) and others have recognized, risk discourse has become central to our understanding of society in late modernity. In one sense, the idea of risk, of a 'risk society', has emerged in response to a belief that modern society is ever more uncertain, contingent, flexible and risky (Turner 1992). However, in terms of epidemiology and other medical and public health discourses, risk refers to something which can be measured (Peterson and Lupton 1996). Thus, it might be argued that there are two broad ways of conceptualizing risk: the 'scientific' approach emerging from epidemiology and the 'lived' or socially experienced dimension (Gifford 1986). Epidemiologists do not work directly with 'risky' bodies. Instead they deal with abstract statistics and often avoid having to face real people or their circumstances. In contrast, lay people demonstrate greater flexibility by sometimes embracing official accounts of health and illness and health risks, while at other times ignoring or resisting these definitions in order to suit their own experiences and make sense within their own circumstances.

Lay and traditional epidemiologies are not mutually exclusive. Lay epidemiological knowledges are as socially constructed as traditional epidemiological facts and people's notions of being 'at risk' are usually shaped by epidemiological understandings of risk. It is important to recognize that while epidemiologists are trained in the scientific 'way of seeing', they too develop their knowledge via their personal experiences. After all, epidemiologists are laypeople first and cannot deny the impact that wider society has upon the ways in which they view the world. While the question of how laypeople define health and illness has emerged as a central theme within the social sciences (Pill and Stott 1982; Blaxter 1983; Williams 1983; Calnan 1987; Eyles and Donovan 1990; Litva and Eyles 1994) it remains marginalized information, scarcely recognized beyond sociology as legitimate knowledge. Despite most health professionals recognizing that laypeople have ideas about the causes of ill health, these ideas tend to be viewed as interesting but irrational.

Davison *et al.* (1992) originally used the phrase **lay epidemiology** to denote the understanding of health risk held by non-medically-qualified people based upon the observation of their own and other people's health experiences. Frankel *et al.* (1991) state that lay epidemiology is the process by which a person interprets health risk through routine observation and discussion of illness and death in personal networks and the public arena, as well as from formal and informal evidence arising from other sources such as television and magazines. People often move between 'official' and lay accounts of the causes of illness without upsetting their own equilibrium. They can hold beliefs about the value of responsible healthy behaviour and the importance of good mental attitudes on one hand and the concepts of fate, luck and inevitability on the other. Pollock (1988) has found that stress has become dominant in most people's understandings of the aetiology of illness and in the ways in which they think about their lives. Several studies have indicated that people living in western societies perceive health as a personal responsibility requiring 'good' health behaviour such as increased physical activity, reducing fat intake and not smoking (Herzlich and Pierret 1987; Lupton 1996). Davison *et al.* (1992) showed that among laypeople there was the belief that a good lifestyle could contribute to good health, although it appears that laypeople may completely ignore or modify such definitions at times in the pursuit of their own interests and goals. Alongside these beliefs were forces external to the individual such as luck, fate and heredity, which also influence whether an individual defines him or herself as ill (Cornwell 1984; Crawford 1984; Calnan 1987; Litva and Eyles 1994; Blaxter 1997).

Wiles's study of heart attack patients demonstrated that, after coming to terms with the shock of the event, patients' trust in 'official' accounts of cause and recovery diminished over time as they turned to evidence from personal observations (Wiles 1998). While they were willing initially to comply with recommended lifestyle changes, over time many returned to their initial behaviours as they began to distrust the actual value gained by changing their lifestyle. Davison *et al.* (1992) also found that, while people view lifestyle change as a health-enhancing action that can reduce the risk of heart disease, at the same time they are aware of the difficulties of practising orthodox preventative health behaviour as well as the random nature of disease distribution. It is also evident that different considerations apply if the individual risk is so small or long term that its assessment is beyond the experience of the individual, or where the changes in behaviour required have negative social or economic effects.

Studies of attitude and opinion in the UK show that ignorance of the main health risk behaviours amongst individuals is rare (Calnan 1987; Blaxter 1990). What is also apparent is that people do not believe that the causes of health and illness lie either totally outside or totally inside the realm of individual control. Most people know that certain behaviours, such as smoking cigarettes, are bad for one's health; however, while these behaviours are attributed values by individuals, it would be wrong to assume that people feel that what is bad for you will always cause death or illness. Rose (cited in Davison *et al.* 1992) suggests that one of the problematic outcomes of public health initiatives based upon traditional epidemiology is thus the **prevention paradox**. This results when lots of people are persuaded to make changes in their lifestyle thereby reducing the overall population risk, while few individuals actually gain any obvious personal benefit. Such simplistic initiatives overlook or play down the complexities of the interactions of personal behaviour and genetic susceptibility. Laypeople are well aware that disease is multifactorial and randomly distributed. From their daily experiences they can see that social factors such as housing, income and occupation can impact upon health. They are also aware that age and sex can increase or negate potential risks. In Backett and Davison's (1992) study, many young people felt that they could drink in excess, smoke or eat 'junk food' without any risk to their health owing to their youth and regular participation in exercise. Older informants, however, did accept some deterioration in health status and felt that they had to modify such behaviours accordingly.

The tension that exists between epidemiological evidence and personal experience is a result of the 'mapping' of data collected from aggregated populations onto the unique trajectory of a single life (Gifford 1986). Put simply, there is a tendency to assume that the results of traditional epidemiological studies apply uniformly and equally to all people. From a scientific perspective a simple grasp of confidence intervals would counter this misconception. From a lay perspective, people observe that many who appear as definite cancer or heart attack recipients, in that they smoke excessively, are overweight and drink excessively, may live to a ripe old age while the most careful person may suddenly die young of a heart attack (Davison *et al.* 1992; Lupton 1996). Because of such experiences many people reject evidence based on traditional epidemiology. Based upon their own observations, they lose trust in 'official' accounts.

Lay knowledge can enhance our understanding of the relationship between social circumstances and individual behaviour (Popay and Williams 1996). Graham's (1987) study of smoking patterns amongst women living in poor material circumstances demonstrated how living in difficult circumstances causes them consciously to use cigarettes to cope with the stresses and strains of daily life. This was not because they were unaware of the risks of smoking behaviour but simply because coping with the poor circumstances in which they lived was of greater importance than the perceived potential risk of smoking cigarettes. There is little attempt by public health and epidemiology to take lay knowledge into account. If research is done, it is usually to explore why laypeople use different types of explanations or do not comply with recommended treatments, rather than to inform understandings about the causes of ill health.

Conclusion

We have explored two different dimensions to the limits of traditional epidemiology. We have argued that, while the biomedical approach has been a useful tool in the quest to eradicate illness in our society, it is seriously limited in its ability to grasp both the causes and consequences of illness. If epidemiological research is to develop more robust and holistic explanations for the patterns of illness and health in society, it must first look critically at its epistemological assumptions and then utilize and build upon critical contextualized understandings and lay perceptions of health, illness and risk. If there is to be a more critical approach as well as the utilization of lay knowledge, innovative methods will have to be explored and other disciplines involved. We do not argue that 'professional expertise' or traditional epidemiology should be devalued. However, there is a need to be more flexible in our 'ways of knowing' and to be aware of the ways in which knowledge, both lay and professional, is constructed.

It would be unfair to suggest that the concerns raised in this chapter are unacknowledged within epidemiology. The operationalization of the approaches that we have discussed requires an awareness of the social, cultural and political context within which disease happens and an understanding of lay interpretations of the experience and aetiology of disease. There is growing evidence that the skills in qualitative methods and sociological analysis necessary to achieve this operationalization are now recognized as necessary to the understanding of disease epidemiology. We conclude by recommending that traditional epidemiology should be practised alongside critical and lay perspectives in order to create a more holistic epidemiological approach that takes account of both social structure and lay knowledge. We suggest that it is only through the incorporation of critical and lay epidemiologies into traditional epidemiological 'ways of knowing' that we will begin to develop a broader and more accurate understanding of the mechanisms by which patterns of health and illness emerge.

Summary

- The study of health and illness is a subject that requires multiple perspectives and multiple approaches. As currently practised, it is often poorly equipped to explain the role of wider social processes in the patterning of health and illness. As epidemiology has moved away from these public health origins, it has increasingly become focused upon the explanatory power of its methods rather than upon the people it studies. The result is an exclusion of the contexts in which disease happens, unless they are immediately measurable, and the voices of those people whose social conditions threaten their health and place them at risk of illness and disease.

- Critical epidemiology seeks to move towards an approach that takes account of the social structures and processes within which ill health originates. It seeks to explain how contextual issues impact upon individual-level risk behaviours. Such work not only recognizes the role(s) played by, for example, multinational companies in the production and consumption of health and illness, it also recognizes the importance of other social processes and forces which structure an individual's ability to make choices.

- Disease and illness are culturally constructed concepts interpreted through both lay and biomedical knowledge systems. Lay and traditional epidemiologies are not mutually exclusive. Lay epidemiological knowledges are as socially constructed as traditional epidemiological facts, and people's notions of being 'at risk' are usually shaped by epidemiological understandings of risk. Despite most health professionals recognizing that laypeople have ideas about the causes of ill health, these ideas tend to be viewed as interesting but irrational. Lay knowledge can enhance our understanding of the relationship between social circumstances and individual health.

Further reading

Davison, C., Frankel, S. and Davey Smith, G. (1992) Lay epidemiology and the prevention paradox: the implication of coronary candidacy for health education, *Sociology of Health and Illness*, 13: 1–19.

Jones, K. and Moon, G. (1987) *Health, Disease and Society*. London: Routledge, chapter 9.

Lupton, D. (1997) *Medicine as Culture*. London: Sage.

Pearce, N. (1996) Traditional epidemiology, modern epidemiology, and public health, *American Journal of Public Health*, 86: 678–83.

Peterson, A. and Lupton, D. (1996) *The New Public Health: Health and Self in the Age of Risk*. London: Sage.

Susser, M. (1996) Choosing a future for epidemiology, *American Journal of Public Health*, 86: 668–73.

Syme, S. (1996) To prevent disease: the need for a new approach, in D. Blane, E. Brunner and R. Wilkinson (eds) *Health and Social Organization: Towards a Health Policy for the 21st Century*. London: Routledge.

Activities

1 Try contextualizing some of the common diseases or health problems you encounter in your everyday practice as a health professional, or as an individual interested in health matters. Take the condition you are interested in and place it in its social, political and cultural context. How can health professionals try to take account of these contexts in everyday practice?

2 Talk to some friends who are not involved in health work about a disease that interests you. Try to get them to focus their accounts on what they think causes the disease. Collect a few different accounts and compare and contrast them with the received clinical view of the disease. If you have access to people with that disease and they are willing to talk, seek their accounts as well. Are there any further differences?

THE PRACTICE OF EPIDEMIOLOGY

This final chapter examines the day-to-day application of epidemiology in operational and strategic planning in the UK NHS. The chapter draws upon two of the authors' experiences working within one (district) health authority.[1] One author (PI) was district epidemiologist for five years and another (GM) was seconded as an epidemiological and research methods consultant. The chapter first considers a range of routine work undertaken on an annual basis and then looks at examples of project-based work of a strategic nature. Much of the routine work is undertaken annually and supports and informs a range of planning and evaluation activities. It draws upon many of the routine data sources identified in Chapter 3 and uses a variety of techniques described elsewhere. The examples of project-based work represent a variety of activities and demonstrate that epidemiological research is not confined to academia but is central to the commissioning of health care.

Annual milestones

Much day-to-day epidemiological work derives from statutory requirements, which are placed on health authorities by the Department of Health (DoH, through the NHS Executive). These requirements are related to the annual planning/performance monitoring cycle. The case study outlined

---

1 The comments and views expressed in this chapter are those of PI and GM and do not
  necessarily represent those of Portsmouth and South East Hampshire Health Authority.

here is based on one author's experiences and relates to the 1997/98 financial year. The implementation of the White Paper on the NHS (DoH 1997) may have altered the nature and timing of the activities described and resulted in some changes to the names of various elements of the planning/performance monitoring cycle, but the broad framework, which we discuss, has remained similar.

There are four key drivers to the annual planning and monitoring cycle from an epidemiologist's perspective:

- *Priorities and Planning Guidance* and the epidemiological data requirements of the corporate contract between the health authority and the NHS Executive (NHSE).
- The statutory responsibility to provide data for the NHS **Common Information Core**.
- The provision of background data and decision-making information to formal health authority meetings.
- The requirement on the director of public health to produce an annual report on the health of the local population.

Each of these is considered, together with work associated with them. There is also consideration of data sources, methods and technique used by the district epidemiologist in undertaking tasks associated with the annual planning/monitoring cycle.

Priorities and Planning Guidance and the corporate contract

The *National Priorities and Planning Guidance* sets out the aims of the government's health policy. It can be found on the World Wide Web at http://www.doh.gov.uk/coinh.htm. It indicates the predicted pressures that require management and also the areas for development that will need attention during the forthcoming financial year. The guidance notes set out the national context for planning whilst also acknowledging the need to accommodate local needs and circumstances. Each health authority agrees an annual plan, known as the corporate contract, with the appropriate NHS Executive Regional Office. These corporate contracts normally reflect national guidance and identify local milestones, objectives and criteria for success. The performance of health authorities is judged on the basis of these corporate contracts.

During the early autumn the health authority produces a consultation document to seek local views on priorities for developments. It sets out issues to be addressed throughout the forthcoming financial year and will typically reflect a mix of national and local priorities. The choice of priorities is determined partly by local and national debate, but is also informed by the results of epidemiological studies and other research evidence. Lobbying and media pressure also have a role in contributing to and shaping national priorities.

The local consultation document makes use of a range of epidemiological information. Key demographic data and information on household composition are used to describe and profile the health authority's local population using the techniques and approaches discussed in Chapter 3.

Raw data are drawn from the routine sources discussed in Chapter 2. The UK census is a key source of data used for this task (Dale and Marsh 1993). Understanding future population needs is also important in planning services and requires making use of population estimates and population projections. Many local authorities in England and Wales produce population estimates and projections for small areas known as electoral wards (Rees 1994). These estimates complement health-authority-level population estimates produced by the ONS and other government departments (OPCS 1992a, b).

In some instances the consultation document might also detail proposals for new local service developments. Data from a range of primary and secondary sources are sometimes utilized to identify potential need for the new service development under consideration. Data on disease incidence and prevalence in the local population might be obtained by applying the results of other surveys to the local population and estimating expected levels of need. The health surveys mentioned in Chapter 3 provide some potential sources of data for this type of approach. Literature searches can be used to identify studies for conditions not covered by the routine data sources (see Chapter 8). Much of the literature on assessing health needs contains prevalence and incidence rates for particular conditions as well as details of effective interventions (Stevens and Raftery 1994). In some cases, proposed service developments will involve some expansion of existing services, and descriptive epidemiology can also help provide evidence of need in these cases. Finally, comparative analysis may be used to highlight differences in service levels and disease prevalence or incidence between different areas. An important element in a health authority case for a development is the recognition of initiatives that have worked in 'similar' areas. The ONS 'area classification' is a valuable means of identifying like areas for making such comparisons (Wallace and Denham 1996).

The Common Information Core

The Common Information Core (CIC) is a range of information required and collected by the NHS Executive to support and facilitate the planning and monitoring cycle nationally. The data collected include activity and financial information against which local commissioning intentions and plans (the performance contract) are monitored and analysed. Additionally, the CIC is used by government health departments to evaluate the implementation of key policies and to brief ministers, to provide purchasers and providers with information on performance, and to inform Parliament and the general public.

Health authorities are required to submit a number of data returns on either an annual or a quarterly basis and these are collated and subsequently used to create the CIC. Data returns include routine epidemiological information relating to *Health of the Nation* targets (for example, coronary heart disease mortality rates and childhood immunization coverage). Information from the *Public Health Common Data Set* is often extracted when making returns as this contains rates rather than raw numbers of cases. Hospital activity data are also collected but are restricted

Table 10.1 Reports to formal health authority meetings, 1997/98 (case study health authority)

Month	Topic/report
1997 September	• Annual health report
	• *Health of the Nation* monitoring
	• Cervical screening
November	• Clinical audit
	• Health alliances
1998 January	• *Public Health Common Data Set* and outcome indicators
	• Breast screening
March	• Clinical effectiveness framework
	• Communicable diseases
May	• Immunization and vaccination

to certain acute procedures and hospital episodes associated with specific conditions. The nature and availability of hospital episode statistics and some of the issues of access to data have been described in Chapter 3.

Formal health authority meetings

Formal health authority meetings are generally held every two months. Part of these meetings is open to the general public and includes presentation of a document on the health of the local population known as the monitoring report. Separate agenda items are used to address significant local issues. There are a number of issues on which the public health department reports throughout the year either in the monitoring report or as a separate agenda item (Table 10.1). The reports make extensive use of many of the data sources and methods described in earlier chapters and are used to identify variations in health outcomes (both spatially and temporally) and chart progress towards meeting strategic aims.

The annual report on the health of the population

Health authority directors of public health medicine are required by statute to produce annual reports on the health status of their local populations (DHSS 1988a). The intention of such reports is to highlight the important health issues relating to the local population, make recommendations for health improvements, and to report progress made since the last annual report. Secondary data sources provide a relatively fast and cost-effective option for commenting on the health status of the local population. As discussed in Chapter 2, it is important to recognize that these 'routine' data sources were originally collected for some primary purpose and their secondary use might be invalid and problematic.

Population characteristics are presented by drawing extensively on the findings of the national census to identify demographic and socioeconomic characteristics of the population (Dale and Marsh 1993). Modern computer software makes it relatively straightforward to analyse population sub-groups and compare subareas (wards or districts) located within health authority areas (Davies 1995; Kinnear and Gray 1997). Alternatively, census enumeration districts (EDs) or wards can be aggregated to user-defined localities (Rhind 1983). Some health authorities have enlisted academic consultants to design local service boundaries (Twigg 1990; Bullen *et al.* 1995; Kivell *et al.* 1990).

The annual reports will typically include some consideration of lifestyle and its effects on health. Where available, data are taken from a local cross-sectional (or possibly prospective cohort) health and lifestyle surveys. These are used to present prevalence, and occasionally incidence, data on major risk factors such as smoking, excessive alcohol consumption, poor diet and lack of exercise. Local surveys will typically include an area identifier (postcode or electoral ward) for respondents thereby enabling geographical patterns to be described. Depending upon the content of local surveys (for example, questions asked, survey design and characteristics of respondents), comparisons can be made with data from other surveys, whether national or for other areas.

The annual report will pay particular attention to patterns of mortality and the impact of different conditions on the local population. The health of the local population may be compared with that of other regions and national data using rates. Variations in health outcomes might be explored using ecological analysis of mortality (or morbidity) rates and local population characteristics derived from the census such as deprivation or unemployment status (Townsend *et al.* 1988). For the most part these studies will be cross-sectional. Where possible, however, use will be made of local studies with case-comparison designs and reference will certainly be made to national studies on relevant topics. Typically, annual health reports focus on a particular aspect of health, a care group or a topical condition and this provides an opportunity to collate morbidity data as well as local and national research studies on the focus issue. As discussed in Chapter 3, morbidity data are harder to access than mortality data, and service activity data are often used as a proxy measure. In seeking to understand the impact of a particular condition or the services used by a care group, the opportunity is taken to collect data from all local service providers. This will include NHS providers (acute and community trusts), private hospitals, the voluntary sector, social services, and local authority education and housing departments. Data on service provision can be compared and contrasted with expected levels by applying consultation rates from national data sources (hospital episode statistics and *Morbidity Statistics from General Practice*).

In addition to collecting, collating and presenting data, the annual report requires the epidemiologist to draw upon local knowledge to interpret the findings presented. Much of the work described above draws on secondary data and requires a good understanding of the range of sources, their strengths and weaknesses and appropriateness for the study under consideration. There will also be a need to understand the strengths and weaknesses of different study designs and, as annual reports increasingly seek to promote evidence-based health care, this will extend to a requirement to interpret and evaluate the quality of evidence in favour of the different interventions available to address the health needs of the population.

Project-based work

Perhaps the greatest opportunity to deploy the full range of analytical techniques and presentation tools used by the district epidemiologist is provided by project work. The examples described here are intended to illustrate the use of both secondary data and the primary collection of data. They are again drawn from one author's (PI) experiences working as a district epidemiologist.

Resource allocation

The method used by Department of Health to allocate resources to health authorities is one that has evolved over a number of years. In 1975 the Resource Allocations Working Party (RAWP) investigated ways of distributing resources that more closely reflected need rather than historical funding patterns (Jones and Moon 1987; Mohan 1995). The RAWP formula resulted and was subsequently reviewed in the late 1980s with a view to improving the accuracy with which it measured relative need (DHSS 1988b). This led in 1989 to a revised capitation funding formula in which the resident population was weighted for the cost of treating patients of different ages (the age–cost curve), relative need (using standardized mortality ratios as a proxy) and for a simple market forces factor. The weightings were reviewed in 1993 by a team from York University (Carr-Hill et al. 1994). Resources are currently allocated to health authorities using population-level characteristics, typically measured on a geographical basis and derived from the census and mortality statistics.

During 1997/98 many health authorities were beginning to investigate the potential use of the national funding formula for allocating resources to GP practices within a health authority (Carr-Hill et al. 1997). During this time one of the authors (PI) joined a regional technical group investigating this issue and brought to the group specialist knowledge of statistical methods and appropriate data sources. The regional technical group's main concern was to determine the validity of applying the capitation funding formula at the sub-health-authority level to GP practice populations. The main issue considered was the appropriateness of the methodology and the reliability of data sources for small populations based on patient lists rather than geographically defined administrative areas. The health authority subsequently adopted the recommendations of the technical group and joint work was undertaken with a consultancy firm to develop a model for allocating resources to GP practices within the district.

The development of health strategies

A key role for epidemiologists working in health authority settings is the development of health strategies to aid the commissioning process. These are usually condition-specific though they may have a care group focus. A health strategy sets out the populations' expected health care needs for a particular condition under consideration and also identifies effective treatments to meet those needs. The approach taken often follows that set out in Stevens and Raftery's (1994) guide to health needs assessment (see also Chapter 8). The basic descriptive epidemiology approach outlined in Chapter 4 provides a framework for development. The key activities are:

- deciding upon the issue to be investigated;
- estimating the size of the health care problem;
- identifying geographical and temporal variations in the problem;
- assessing demographic and socioeconomic variations relevant to the problem;
- identifying and enumerating the risk factors associated with individuals;
- searching for evidence that suggests effective interventions to treat, prevent and diagnose individuals.

Local health surveys to identify disease incidence and prevalence are often not routinely available and would be prohibitively expensive to undertake. Estimates can, however, be generated by 'projecting' results from other areas onto the local population. Local demographic data can be obtained from the census, and population estimates and projections can be used in conjunction with prevalence and incidence rates identified from surveys undertaken elsewhere. Applying national rates to the local population figures will provide a crude estimate of the likely numbers affected in the local population. Clearly, the more similar the survey area and the local population the better the estimate will be. Multilevel modelling techniques can be used to refine the estimates by adjusting for differences in the compositions of the two areas (Twigg *et al.* 2000).

An analysis of the availability and use of local services is likely to be included. Simple dot maps (Cliff and Haggett 1988) provide a potentially powerful presentation of the location of services, particularly when complemented with population details and transport links. Data on the current levels of service use are required to provide a baseline and to highlight variations in the use of those services in terms of different groups within the population. Variations in service use might exist for different age, sex or ethnic groups and be the result of differing referral patterns and differences in accessibility to services (Joseph and Phillips 1984). Such analysis may also inform local audit work and help to assess whether inappropriate procedures are being undertaken.

Mental health needs assessment

All health authorities have limited resources and this means that opportunities for developmental work, and especially for primary data collection, are uncommon but enthusiastically greeted. A multidisciplinary and cross-organizational mental health needs assessment group recognized the requirement to better identify mental health needs in the primary care setting and in particular to inform the allocation of staff resources to GP practices. A study was designed in which ten practices were surveyed (two being selected from each of five 'deprivation' groups) and the level of psychiatric morbidity assessed using a self-completed questionnaire with results being confirmed through examination of GP notes.

GP practices were grouped using the Jarman underprivileged area (UPA) index (Jarman 1983, 1984; Senior 1991). UPA scores for enumeration districts were calculated using census data and standard statistical software. The GP–patient register extracted from the health authority's information system was then used to derive GP practice-based patient lists by postcode. The postcodes were matched to census enumeration districts using the ONS postcode-to-ED look-up table (Martin 1995). A practice score for the UPA index was then derived using ED UPA scores weighted according to the practice populations and combined to each practice. Analysis of the survey data and assistance in interpreting the findings were undertaken jointly between the public health department and an academic (GM) (Moon et al. 1998).

A further element of the mental health needs assessment work was the development of a register of severely mentally ill residents of the health authority. The intentions of this work were to promote improved collaborative working across different agencies and to better understand levels of local psychiatric morbidity in terms of both individual patient characteristics and residential location. Community health care and social services mental health teams were initially invited to identify clients with a severe mental illness. Individual details including age, sex, GP details and a personal identifier were requested. Managerial support for the project was agreed and confidentiality was ensured by storing the data at the health authority using a secure database application developed by the public health department's epidemiology team.

The collected returns were then entered into the computerized database and a list of people with severe mental health problems in contact with the range of statutory agencies was produced for each GP practice. GPs were then asked to validate these lists. The response rate for validating was poor and reduced the value of the database; however, some interesting preliminary results were produced. These were useful in identifying patients who were known only to a few service providers. It should also be noted that there were definitional problems in agreeing what constituted severe mental illness across all the professional groups involved. The original intention was for the register to become the basis of an ongoing operational system to improve patient co-ordination between service providers. In practice, as is often the case, limited resources and changing agendas have meant that the results of the project were not fully exploited.

Other development work

Hospital activity data (finished consultant episode statistics) include some clinical information that can be usefully analysed. It includes the patient's diagnosis, the speciality of their consultant and, where appropriate, details of operative procedure. In many instances, however, analysing hospital activity data by speciality leads to ambiguous comparisons as patients might be treated under different specialists in different areas, and speciality level groupings are very broadly defined. At the other extreme, diagnostic codes and individual procedure codes are too numerous and provide too many categories for many comparative purposes. Healthcare Resource Groups (HRGs) provide a manageable number of groupings and provide an improved basis for data analysis (Sanderson *et al.* 1998). They also enable a better appreciation of the range of conditions and treatments which are involved in the linked episodes of care which cumulatively make up many individuals' experiences of hospital. Understanding this **casemix** is important if health care commissioning is to be effective.

Levels of food-and-hygiene-related notifiable diseases have long been a area of health authority concern (Salisbury and Begg 1996). During the case study period, work was initiated to validate notifications received via ONS (and originally sent by doctors to the local Proper Officer). Data from the Public Health Laboratory Service (PHLS) were used as a benchmark against which notifiable cases were validated and was important in evaluating data quality. Using the more robust validated database, information was used to focus activities on the prevention of infectious diseases (for example, improving food hygiene). The project was also invaluable in encouraging joint working with local authority staff.

High rates of teenage pregnancy were another area of concern. A multiagency project was established to investigate further the patterns of teenage pregnancies and to devise a research strategy for investigating teenagers' needs regarding the practice of 'safe sex'. The project also sought to learn about young pregnant women's experiences. The background for this work was set by a descriptive ecological study that made use of routine data on births, conceptions and abortions along with basic demographic information. Mapping techniques (Cliff and Haggett 1988) were appropriate for this work and provided a valuable means of highlighting variations in pregnancy within the health authority and in developing possible hypotheses. The survey methods described in Chapter 2 were then used to test these hypotheses in the field. This work is ongoing but is yielding valuable information to direct the development of local services for teenagers.

Mapping provides a powerful means of presenting health data, and many health authorities have invested in software for doing this (Gould 1992). Two of the authors have been involved in projects to produce a series of community health atlases (Portsmouth and South East Hampshire Health Authority 1990, 1996). These contain maps of births, morbidity and disability, mortality, demography, socioeconomic characteristics, lifestyle, housing, and health service utilization. The atlases have provided key reference material for local health and social care organizations through a thorough description of epidemiological patterns within the health authority area.

Conclusion

Many of the projects presented in this chapter provide good examples of local collaborative work involving a number of health organizations, voluntary bodies and local authority representatives. Collaborative work should become more commonplace as health improvement programmes become developed as part of the 'new, modern, dependable NHS' (DoH 1997). The projects described have tended to reflect prevailing local priorities and policy issues. It will be evident that much of the work is relatively straight-forward. In terms of 'doing epidemiology', the focus is very much towards routine data and the cross-sectional design. Only in project work do the more sophisticated designs enter the scene; nor is there much about critical or lay epidemiology. This picture may, however, be atypical and it is certainly changing as, on the one hand, lay and critical knowledge are recognized as essential to effective health promotion and, on the other hand, evidence-based health care draws increasingly on the skills of epidemiologists and requires familiarity with more advanced approaches.

The epidemiological techniques and approaches identified throughout this book have made a major contribution to practical deployment of epidemiological knowledge both locally and nationally. They are also important for routine operational and strategic policy related work. Descriptive epidemiological techniques are used to identify disease patterns and the generation of hypotheses about their causes. Analytical observational methods enable risk factors associated with diseases to be established, whilst intervention studies allow the effectiveness of health treatments to be assessed. This concluding chapter illustrates the real world context and application of these epidemiological tools in informing a number of different policy tasks and functions. These include providing an information base for the development of local services, allocating resources to meet health care needs, and identifying and understanding local and national priorities. This chapter has demonstrated that the district epidemiologist's job is varied and interesting. Many of the approaches identified are relevant to a wide range of health and social care professionals and researchers and it is hoped that this book will inspire readers to incorporate epidemiological methods into their work.

Summary

- Much day-to-day epidemiological work derives from statutory requirements placed on health authorities by the Department of Health (through the NHS Executive), for example the requirement on the director of public health to produce an annual report on the health of the local population.

- Understanding future population health needs is important in planning services and requires making use of population estimates and population projections and data on disease incidence and prevalence. Applying the results of other surveys to the local population can be used to estimate expected levels of need.

- While the day-to-day application of epidemiology may appear to focus on descriptive and cross-sectional studies, analytical studies are increasingly relevant in view of their use in the development of evidence-based health care.

Further reading

Beaglehole, R., Bonita, R. and Kjellström, T. (1993) *Basic Epidemiology*.
Geneva: WHO.
DoH (Department of Health) (annual) *On the State of the Public Health*.
London: The Stationery Office.

Activities

1 Every year health authorities produce annual public health reports. There
is also a national report called *On the State of the Public Health*. Get hold
of a copy of your local report and also the national one: your NHS or
university library should be able to help. Read both reports critically
and ask yourself what sort of epidemiology is in evidence and note the
use of the different perspectives outlined in this book. Ask yourself
what the implications of the two reports are for your own practice as a
health professional.

2 We have concluded this book with a sort of diary concerning epidemiological activities in a health authority setting. Try to construct a similar
record of your own typical year, noting when you have encounters with
epidemiology.

APPENDIX: INFERENTIAL STATISTICS

Inferential techniques are the branch of statistical methods that use the characteristics of a sample to make inferences about a population. To be able to understand the concepts behind them, a first point of reference is the normal curve frequency distribution described in the text. This is a bell-shaped symmetrical curve whose peak represents the frequency found at the average and median values.

In a perfectly normal curve, because the shape is symmetrical there are an equal number of observations on either side of the central value or average, and it therefore follows that 50 per cent of the observations fall either side of the average. An alternative way of expressing this is that the chance of obtaining an observation which is higher than the average is 50 per cent and that of obtaining one which is lower than the average is also 50 per cent (or a probability of 0.5).

The normal curve can also be described in terms of its standard deviation. The standard deviation indicates the average difference of all values around the mean. In a perfectly normal curve, 68 per cent of the values are found within 1 standard deviation of either side of the mean; 95 per cent of the values will be within almost 2 standard deviations (1.96 to be exact) and 99 per cent of the values will fall within approximately 2.5 standard deviations. These statements may be a little difficult to visualize, but if height is used to illustrate them then it may be easier to understand. If it is assumed, for example, that average height is 66 inches and that the standard deviation is 4 inches, then 68 per cent of the population will be between 62 and 70 inches (that is, 1 standard deviation above and below the mean). Likewise, approximately 95 per cent of the people will be between 58 and 74 inches and 99 per cent between 54 and 78 inches.

If an infinite number of similar sized samples are taken from a population, then the mean of these results will equate with the population mean and the distribution of the sample means will be normal in appearance. Furthermore, the standard deviation of this distribution, known as the *standard error*, is given by the standard deviation of the sampling distribution divided by the square root of the sample size. Knowing the standard error enables the researcher to estimate how far into the tails of the normal curve a particular sample value occurs. If it is more than 3 standard errors away from the population average, then the researcher knows that such a value would occur only one time in 100 by chance – remember that 99 per cent of values occur within 3 standard deviations of the mean.

It is common in non-clinical epidemiological research to use a cut-off value of 95 per cent as the decision point for such 'significance'. This is often referred to as the p-value and expressed as $p < 0.05$. This means that the researcher will accept the significance of a research value if it is expected to occur by chance less than 5 times out of 100. Note that this is less strict than $p < 0.01$ or $p < 0.001$. Testing for significance at the 95 per cent level therefore involves calculating a standard error and assessing whether an observed test statistic is more than 1.96 standard errors away from a reference value. Similarly, the confidence interval is the *credible* interval around the given value as supported by the data. A 95 per cent confidence interval will be plus or minus 1.96 standard errors around an observed value. With a large sample there will be a narrow interval, and with a small sample there will be a large interval.

GLOSSARY

Aetiology: cause(s).

Analytical designs: studies which aim to identify associations between a disease and possible causes. They test hypotheses.

Attributable risk: an estimate of the potential for disease prevention. In particular, it is used when assessing how much of the incidence of disease can be prevented if the exposure is reduced to zero.

Attrition: the loss of study respondents as they are followed over time. A particular problem in experimental and cohort studies.

Case-comparison (or case-control) studies: begin with diseased cases and healthy comparisons ('controls') and search for differences between the two groups in terms of past exposure to risk factors.

Casemix: the range of conditions and treatments that are involved in the linked episodes of care which cumulatively make up many individuals' experiences of hospital.

Census: a total enumeration of the population and a selection of its characteristics.

Chronic-disease epidemiology: the study of conditions such as heart disease and cancers that are overwhelmingly the major killers in western society.

Clinical effectiveness: the extent to which a treatment, procedure, therapy or service achieves its intended purpose for its target patients.

Clinical epidemiology: epidemiological work that focuses on disease causes which can be found in the internal mechanics of the body.

Clinical iceberg: the fact that most disease is self-treated, ignored or undiagnosed.

Cochrane Library: a computerized database that can be searched for systematic reviews, clinical trials and other evidence-based health care information.

Coding: giving numerical codes to responses in a survey or other data collection exercise.

Cohort studies: the monitoring of exposed and non-exposed subjects through time to compare their respective chances of the development of disease.

Common Information Core (CIC): a range of information required and collected by the NHS Executive to support and facilitate the national planning and monitoring cycle.

Communicable-disease epidemiology: the study of the causes of diseases that can be spread or 'caught'. Such diseases are less common than they once were in the West, but communicable disease epidemiology retains an importance in the developing world and has continued relevance to the West in the study of AIDS/HIV and resurgent tuberculosis.

Community epidemiology: work in which emphasis is placed on disease surveillance and occurrence in real-world settings, screening and the implementation of community-based interventions.

Community trials: experimental studies in which a group or population is subject to a particular intervention and is compared with a group which does not receive the intervention.

Confidence interval: a range of values likely, with a specified degree of certainty, to contain the true population figure for a variable drawn from a sample study.

Confounding: a variable (usually unrecognized) that influences the observed relationship between an exposure and outcome. Confounding variables are related to both exposure and outcome and need to be controlled for.

Continuous data: numerical values on an ordered scale with real or arbitrary zero points. Best understood as all data which are neither ordinal (1st, 2nd, 3rd and so on) or nominal (present/absent; red/white/blue and so on).

Control: in analysis, a variable which is used to 'allow for' another variable; that is, to test for a confounder.

Control group: the group in an experimental design that is not exposed to an intervention; also sometimes confusingly used to refer to the comparison group in case-comparison studies (that is, the group which does not experience the outcome).

Co-variation: exposure and outcome should co-vary over space and time if they are causally related. If air pollution is a cause of bronchitis then an increase in air pollution should be associated with an increase in bronchitis and highly polluted parts of the country should have a high incidence of bronchitis.

Critical appraisal: structured reading and analysis of epidemiological or health services research according to published guidelines.

Critical epidemiology: places an emphasis on the social and power relations that shape disease definition and disease causation.

Cross-sectional (or prevalence) studies: a particular type of descriptive study. A cross-sectional study involves selecting a sample of subjects and then determining the distribution of exposure and disease within that sample.

Cumulative incidence: *see* Incidence proportion.

Disease determinants: factors or events that are capable of bringing about a change in health.

Dose–response relationship: traditionally applied in randomized clinical trials of new drugs to denote the relationship between the dose and the outcome. Now often extended to the notion that the length or strength of an exposure relates to the severity/extent/duration of an outcome

Double-blind experiment: where neither the patent nor the practitioner knows who has been assigned to a control or intervention group in a randomized clinical trial.

Effect modifier: a variable in an epidemiological causal model which is causal in its own right but also alters the magnitude of the causal effect of another causal variable.

Eligible population: those people who are defined (on the basis of explicit criteria) as being eligible for entry into a study.

Enumeration districts (EDs): small geographical areas for which census data are available.

Epistemological strategy: the way in which a discipline constructs and frames its knowledge base.

Evidence-based health care: the identification of the best and most appropriate ways of treating and managing patients according to available high quality published evidence.

Evidence-based medicine: the use of research evidence, often from epidemiological studies, to ensure that only the most effective procedures are used in disease management.

Experiment of opportunity: *see* Natural experiment.

Experimental (or interventionist) designs: studies in which the investigator intervenes to create the desired situation and to manipulate the causal factor to see what effect it has. Sound experiments involve the random allocation of participants between control and intervention groups. The intervention group is the one which is exposed to the hypothesized causal variable.

External validity: the extent to which the results of a study can be generalized to a wider population.

Finished consultant episodes (FCEs): a measure of the work undertaken by hospital consultants.

Healthcare Resource Groups (HRGs): an approach to grouping hospital episodes of care by diagnosis, procedure and costing. HRGs aim to provide a manageable and coherent number of groupings for further analysis.

Hospital activity data: routinely collected data within hospital settings relating to clinical activity.

Hypothesis: a tentative answer to a research question. A prediction. Usually the basis for a test.

Incidence: the number of new cases of a disease that come into being in a specified population during a specified period of time.

Incidence proportion (or cumulative incidence): the proportion of unaffected individuals who, on average, will contract a disease of interest over a specified period of time.

Incidence rate (IR) (or incidence density): the rapidity with which newly diagnosed disease develops.

Inference: making general predictions on the basis of the analysis of a sample. Usually understood in epidemiology in relation to statistical methods.

Information bias: systematic misclassification.

Interaction: in epidemiological methods, the joint action of two or more exposures impacting upon an outcome (as opposed to the individual impact of an exposure).

Internal validity: the extent to which the results of a study stand up in terms of the design and conduct of the study; the extent to which the study can justifiably be held to have generated its purported results.

International Classification of Disease (ICD): a coding system for causes of death.

Interventionist designs: *see* Experimental designs.

Lay epidemiology: the understanding of health risk held by non-medically-qualified people based upon the observation of their own and other people's health experiences.

Matched design: comparisons chosen to match individual cases for certain important variables such as age and sex.

Mean: the 'average', a measure of level that involves adding up all the values of interest and dividing by the number of values.

MeSH terms (Medical Subject Headings): a thesaurus of nearly 18,000 main subjects that are used to classify articles in the Medline database.

Meta-analysis: a statistical technique used to assemble results from several studies and create a single estimate for a particular health outcome.

Modelling: in statistical analysis, the use of statistical theory to 'control by analysis'. Statistical models 'explain' the variation in an outcome of interest in terms of a set of several exposure factors.

Multivariate analysis: in statistical analysis, taking simultaneous account of the effect of more than two exposures on an outcome.

Natural or quasi-experiment (or experiment of opportunity): the researcher does not deliberately manipulate the supposed causal variable, but attempts to discover real-world situations in which the possibly causal variable has varied and then to observe the effect of these changes on disease outcomes. Not a true experiment and lacking randomization.

Normal curve (or Gaussian curve): a statistically defined ideal frequency distribution which is symmetrical about a single peak (the mean) and bell-shaped.

Notification: medical personnel (in general practice and hospitals) are required to notify cases of certain diseases, mainly infectious diseases, to the local 'proper officer'.

Occupational epidemiology: focuses on the workplace, monitors the levels of disease in the workforce, and looks for causal relations between occupational exposures and subsequent disease.

Odds: the ratio of the probability of dying/becoming ill to the probability of surviving/remaining well.

Panel study: a survey where the same individuals are asked the same questions at successive interviews.

Period prevalence: the proportion of the population recorded as having the disease over a specified time period.

Placebo: an inert treatment with a known lack of effect on disease; administered in a trial in order to isolate the hypothesized causal effect of a treatment under investigation.

Point prevalence: the proportion of a population known to have the disease at a particular time.

Poisson distribution: a statistically defined frequency distribution that describes the occurrence of rare events following a random, rather than systematic process.

Popular epidemiology: *see* Lay epidemiology.

Population estimate: an estimate of the population base between censuses.

Population projection: an extrapolation of population data using known patterns of births, deaths and migration to predict figures.

Population-based prevention: aimed at everybody and concerned with reducing overall levels of risk.

Precision: the ability of a measure to detect change; the degree of absence of random error.

Prevalence: the number of *existing cases* of a disease or health condition in a specific population at some designated time or during some designated time period.

Prevalence studies: *see* Cross-sectional studies.

Prevention paradox: when lots of people are persuaded to make changes in their lifestyle thereby reducing the overall population risk, while few individuals actually gain any obvious personal benefit.

Primary data: data collected directly from the public by a researcher/epidemiologist, for example by a survey.

Prospective design: a study in which data are collected from a defined starting point into the future. The determination of exposure levels at baseline (the present) with subjects being followed for occurrence of disease at some time in the future.

Random sampling: a method of selecting individuals to take part in a survey; individuals have an equal probability of being chosen and are selected from a larger sampling frame using random numbers.

Randomization: assignment of people at random to control or intervention groups in a randomized clinical trial.

Randomized Clinical Trial (RCT): study in which an experimental group is given a new, untried therapy, drug or vaccine, while the control group is given a treatment in current use or no treatment at all.

Recall bias: situations where those with the disease are more likely to recall past exposures.

Reductionist principles: breaking an issue of concern into its component parts. Can work at the expense of understanding context and interactions.

Relative risk: the comparison of the incidence of a disease or condition between a group with a particular attribute or exposure to one without; indicates the magnitude of the increased risk derived from the exposure.

Repeated cross-sectional study: in this sort of study, cross-sections of the population are asked the same questions on different occasions but no attempt is made to sample the same people in each repetition.

Retrospective design: a study that makes use of historical data to determine exposure level at some baseline in the past.

Routine statistics: statistical data which result from regular recorded activity.

Sample: a subset of the population.

Secondary data: data collected and published by others.

Selection bias: occurs when subjects who are selected and participate in a study are different in a systematic way from those excluded from the study.

Selective prevention: is aimed at those at high-risk. In epidemiological terms this requires the ability to screen into separate high- and low-risk groups.

Significance: in statistical analysis, the probability of an event occurring by chance.

Single-blind experiment: a randomized clinical trial in which the patients do not know whether they are in an experimental group receiving treatment or in a control group.

Social construction: the way in which prevailing economic, social and political circumstances frame the understanding of a phenomenon.

Social epidemiology: considers determinants of health and illness that are rooted in the divisions of contemporary society.

Standard deviation: a statistical measure that describes the average spread of all the values around the mean.

Standardization: controlling for the effects of age or other variables on a chosen issue.

Standardized mortality ratio (SMR): the ratio of the actual (or observed) deaths to the expected deaths.

Strata: a set of population subgroups used as distinct sampling bases in a survey.

Study design: strategies for conducting research and gaining information.

Synergistic interaction: interactions in which the independent effects of two or more exposures are enhanced by the presence of the other factors.

Systematic review: a synthesis of evidence published on a chosen topic. The selection of evidence is guided by strict criteria concerning study design quality. Quantitative comparisons of results are usually presented.

Target population: the population to which the results can be applied.

Triangulation: the use of multiple research methods to investigate a question.

Vital events: births, deaths and marriages. The Births, Marriages and Deaths Act 1839 requires their notification to a local registrar.

REFERENCES

Acheson, D. (1967) *Medical Record Linkage*. London: Oxford University Press.

Acheson, D. (1998) *Independent Inquiry into Inequalities in Health* (Acheson Inquiry). London: The Stationery Office.

Alderson, M. (1987) The use of area mortality data, *Population Trends*, 47: 24–33.

Anon. (1994) Population health looking upstream, *The Lancet*, 343: 429–30.

Antman, E., Lau, J., Kupelnick, B., Mosteller, F. and Chalmers, T. (1992) A comparison of results of meta-analyses of randomized control trials and recommendations of clinical experts, *Journal of the American Medical Association*, 268: 240–8.

Armstrong, D. (1993) Public health spaces and the fabrication of identity, *Sociology*, 27: 393–410.

Ashton, J. (ed.) (1994) *The Epidemiological Imagination*. Buckingham: Open University Press.

Backett, K. and Davison, C. (1992) Rational or reasonable? Perceptions of health at different stages of life, *Health Education Journal*, 51(2): 55–9.

Balarajan, R. (1991) Ethnic differences in mortality from ischaemic heart disease and cerebrovascular disease in England and Wales, *British Medical Journal*, 302: 560–4.

Baldwin, A., Acheson, D. and Graham, W. (eds) (1987) *Textbook of Medical Record Linkage*. Oxford: Oxford Medical Publications.

Bassuk, E. (1986) The rest cure: repetition or resolution of Victorian women's conflicts? in S. Suleiman (ed.) *The Female Body in Western Culture: Contemporary Perspectives*. Cambridge: Harvard University Press.

Beck, U. (1996) Risk, society and the provident state, in S. Lash, B. Szerszynski and B. Wynne (eds) *Risk, Environment and Modernity: Towards a New Ecology*. London: Sage.

Black, D. (1984) *Investigation of the Possible Increased Incidence of Cancer in West Cumbria: Report of the Independent Advisory Group*. London: HMSO.

Blaxter, M. (1983) The causes of disease, *Social Science and Medicine*, 17(2): 59–69.

Blaxter, M. (1990) *Health and Lifestyle*. London: Routledge.

Blaxter, M. (1997) Whose fault is it? People's own conceptions of the reasons for health inequalities, *Social Science and Medicine*, 44(6): 747–56.

Bloor, M., Samphier, M. and Prior, L. (1987) Artefact explanations of inequalities in health: an assessment of the evidence, *Sociology of Health and Illness*, 9: 231–64.

Botting, B. (ed.) (1995) *The Health of our Children*, series DS No. 11. London: HMSO.

Britton, M. (1990) *Mortality and Geography: A Review in the Mid-1980s*, OPCS series DS No. 9. London: HMSO.

Brown, M. (1995) Ironies of distance: an ongoing critique of the geographies of AIDS, *Environment and Planning D: Society and Space*, 13: 159–83.

Bryce, C., Curtis, S. and Mohan, J. (1994) Coronary heart disease: trends in spatial inequalities and implications for health care planning in England, *Social Science and Medicine*, 38: 677–90.

Bryman, A. and Cramer, D. (1994) *Quantitative Data Analysis for Social Scientists*. London: Routledge.

Bryman, A. and Cramer, D. (1996) *Quantitative Data Analysis with Minitab*. London: Routledge.

Buck, N., Gershuny, J., Rose, D. and Scott, J. (eds) (1994) *Changing Households*. Colchester: ESRC Research Centre on Micro-social Change, University of Essex.

Bullen, N., Moon, G. and Jones, K. (1995) Defining localities for health planning: a GIS approach, *Social Science and Medicine*, 42: 801–16.

Calnan, M. (1987) *Health and Illness: The Lay Perspective*. London: Tavistock.

Carr-Hill, R., Sheldon, T., Smith, P., Martin, S., Peacock, S. and Hardman, G. (1994) Allocating resources to health authorities: development of a method for small area analysis of use of inpatient services, *British Medical Journal*, 309: 1046–9.

Carr-Hill, R., Hardman, G., Martin, S., Peacock, S., Sheldon, T. and Smith, P. (1997) A new formula for distributing hospital funds in England, *Interfaces*, 27: 53–70.

Caselli, G. (1994) *Long-term Trends in European Mortality*, OPCS Studies on Medical and Population Subjects No. 56. London: HMSO.

CDCP (Centers for Disease Control and Prevention) (1981) Toxic shock syndrome – United States 1970–1980, *MMWR* 30: 26. Quoted in R. Friis and T. Sellers (1996) *Epidemiology for Public Health Practice*. Gaithersburg, MD: Aspen.

Chalmers, I. and Altman, D. (eds) (1995) *Systematic Reviews*. London: BMJ Publishing Group.

Chalmers, I., Enkin, M. and Keirse, M. (eds) (1985) *Effective Care in Pregnancy and Childbirth*. Oxford: Oxford University Press.

Charlton, J. and Murphy, M. (1997) *The Health of Adult Britain 1841–1994*, series DS No. 12. London: The Stationery Office.

Cheadle, A., Wagner, E., Koepsell, T., Kristal, A. and Patrick, D. (1992) Environmental indicators: a tool for evaluating community-based health promotion programs, *American Journal of Preventative Medicine*, 8: 345–50.

Chilvers, C. (1978) Regional mortality 1969–73, *Population Trends*, 11: 16–20.

Clarke, K., Gray, D., Keating, N. and Hampton, J. (1994) Do women with acute myocardial infarction receive the same treatment as men? *British Medical Journal*, 309: 563–6.

Cliff, A. and Haggett, P. (1988) *Atlas of Disease Distributions: Analytical Approaches to Epidemiological Data*. Oxford: Blackwell.

Cochrane, A. (1972) *Effectiveness and Efficiency: Random Reflections on Health Services*. London: Nuffield Provincial Hospital Trust.

Cole, K. (1993) The 1991 local base and small area statistics, in A. Dale and C. Marsh (eds) *The 1991 Census Users' Guide*. London: HMSO.

Committee on Medical Aspects of Radiation in the Environment (1996) *Fourth Report: The Incidence of Cancer and Leukaemia in the Vicinity of the Sellafield Site, West Cumbria: Further Studies and an Update of the Situation Since the Publication of the Black Advisory Group in 1984*. London: HMSO.

Comstock, G. (1979) Association of water hardness and cardiovascular diseases, in E. Agino (ed.) *Geochemistry of Water in Relation to Cardiovascular Disease*. Washington, DC: National Academy of Sciences.

Cornwell, J. (1984) *Hard-earned Lives*. London: Tavistock.

Cox, B. (1995) *HALS Death Data User Guide*. Colchester: ESRC Data Archive, University of Essex.

Cox, B., Blaxter, M., Buckle, A. *et al.* (1987) *Health and Lifestyle Survey, 1984–85*. London: Health Promotion Research Trust.

Craft, A., Openshaw, S. and Birch, J. (1984) Apparent clusters of childhood lymphoid malignancy in Northern England, *The Lancet*, 14 July, 96–7.

Craft, A., Parker, L., Openshaw, S. *et al.* (1993) Cancer in young people in the north of England, 1968–1985: analysis by census wards, *Journal of Epidemiology and Community Health*, 47: 109–15.

Crawford, R. (1984) A critical account of 'health': control, release and the social body, in J. McKinley (ed.) *Issues in the Political Economy of Health Care*. London: Tavistock.

CRD (Centre for Reviews and Dissemination) (1996) *Undertaking Systematic Reviews of Research on Effectiveness: CRD Guidelines for Those Carrying Out or Commissioning*

Reviews, CRD Report No. 4. York: NHS Centre for Reviews and Dissemination, University of York.

Crombie, I. and Davies, H. (1996) *Research in Health Care*. Chichester: John Wiley.

Curtis, S., Eames, M., Ben-Shlomo, Y., Marmot, M., Mohan, J. and Killoran, A. (1993) Geographical differences in CHD mortality in England: implications for local health planning. *Health Education Journal*, 52(2): 72–8.

D'Agostino, R. and Kwan, H. (1995) Measuring effectiveness: what to expect without a randomized control group, *Medical Care*, 33: 95–105.

Dale, A. (1993a) The content of the 1991 census: change and continuity, in A. Dale and C. March (eds) *The 1991 Census User's Guide*. London: HMSO.

Dale, A. (1993b) The OPCS Longitudinal Study, in A. Dale and C. Marsh (eds) *The 1991 Census User's Guide*. London: HMSO.

Dale, A. and Marsh, C. (eds) (1993) *The 1991 Census User's Guide*. London: HMSO.

Davey-Smith, G. and Shipley, M. (1991) Confounding of occupation and smoking: its magnitude and consequences, *Social Science and Medicine*, 32: 1297–300.

Davies, H. (1995) Accessing the data via SASPAC 91, in S. Openshaw (ed.) *Census Users' Handbook*. Cambridge: GeoInformation International.

Davison, C., Frankel, S. and Davey Smith, G. (1992) Lay epidemiology and the prevention paradox: the implication of coronary candidacy for health education, *Sociology of Health and Illness*, 13: 1–19.

Dawber, T., Kannel, W. and Lyell, L. (1993) An approach to longitudinal studies in a community: the Framingham study, *Annals of the New York Academy of Science*, 107: 539–56.

Denham, C. (1993) Outputs from the 1991 Census: an introduction, in A. Dale and C. Marsh (eds) *The 1991 Census Users' Guide*. London: HMSO.

DHSS (Department of Health and Social Security) (1980) *Inequalities in Health: the Report of a Research Working Group Chaired by Sir Douglas Black* (Black Report). London: DHSS.

DHSS (Department of Health and Social Security) (1988a) *Public Health in England. The Report of the Committee of Inquiry into the Future Development of the Public Health Function (Chaired by Sir Donald Acheson)*, (Cm. 289). London: HMSO.

DHSS (Department of Health and Social Security) (1988b). *Review of the Resource Allocation Working Party Formula: Final Report by the NHS Management Board*. London: DHSS.

Diez-Roux, A. (1998) On genes, individuals, society, and epidemiology, *American Journal of Epidemiology*, 148: 1027–32.

Dixon, R., Munro, J., and Silcocks, P. (1997) *The Evidence Based Medicine Workbook: Critical Appraisal for Clinical Problem Solving*. Oxford: Butterworth Heinemann.

DoH (Department of Health) (1992) *Health of the Nation*. London: HMSO.

DoH (Department of Health) (1994) *Coronary Heart Disease: An Epidemiological Overview*. London: HMSO.

DoH (Department of Health) (1995) *Variations in Health: What Can the Department of Health and the NHS Do?* London: DoH.

DoH (Department of Health) (1996) *Research and Development: Towards an Evidence-Based Health*. London: DoH.

DoH (Department of Health) (1997) *The New NHS: Modern, Dependable*, (Cm. 3807). London: The Stationery Office.

DoH (Department of Health) (1998a) *National Service Framework: Coronary Heart Disease: Emerging Findings*. London: DoH.

DoH (Department of Health) (1998b) *Our Healthier Nation*, (Cm. 3852). London: The Stationery Office.

DoH (Department of Health) (1999) *Saving Lives: Our Healthier Nation*, (Cm. 4386). London: The Stationery Office.

DoH (Department of Health) (annual) *On the State of the Public Health*. London: The Stationery Office.

DoH/NIE (Department of Health/National Institute of Epidemiology) (1996) *The Public Health Common Data Set.* London: DoH.

Doll, R. and Hill, A. (1954) The mortality of doctors in relation to their smoking habits, *British Medical Journal*, 1: 1451–5.

Doll, R. and Hill, A. (1964) Mortality in relation to smoking: ten years observations of British doctors, *British Medical Journal*, 1: 1399–410, 1460–7.

Doll, R. and Peto, R. (1976) Mortality in relation to smoking: 20 years of observations on male doctors, *British Medical Journal*, 2: 1525–36.

Doll, R. and Peto, R. (1981) *The Causes of Cancer.* Oxford: Oxford University Press.

Doll, R., Evans, H. and Darby, S. (1994) Paternal exposure not to blame, *Nature*, 367: 678–80.

Douglas, M. and Wildavsky, A. (1982) *Risk and Culture.* Oxford: Blackwell.

Doyal, L. and Epstein, S. (1983) *Cancer in Britain: The Politics of Prevention*, London: Pluto Press.

Drever, F. (1995) *Occupational Health: Decennial Supplement*, series DS No. 10. London: HMSO.

Ekinsmyth, C. (1996) The British longitudinal birth cohort studies: their utility for the study of health and place, *Health and Place*, 2: 15–26.

Elwood, J. (1998) *Critical Appraisal of Epidemiological Studies and Clinical Trials.* Oxford: Oxford University Press.

Epstein, S. (1979) *The Politics of Cancer.* New York: Anchor.

Erickson, B. and Nosanchuk, T. (1992) *Understanding Data.* Buckingham: Open University Press.

Eyles, J. and Donovan, J. (1990) *The Social Effects of Health Policy.* Aldershot: Gower.

Farmer, P. (1992) *AIDS and Accusation: Haiti and the Geography of Blame.* Berkeley: University of California Press.

Farmer, P. (1996) On suffering and structural violence: a view from below, *Daedalus*, Winter: 261–83.

Farmer, R., Miller, D. and Lawrenson, R. (1996) *Lecture Notes on Epidemiology and Public Health Medicine.* Oxford: Blackwell.

Fleck, L. ([1936] 1979) *Genesis and Development of a Scientific Fact.* Chicago: University of Chicago Press.

Foucault, M. (1984) The politics of health in the eighteenth century, in P. Rabinow (ed.) *The Foucault Reader: An Introduction to Foucault's Thought.* New York: Pantheon.

Fox, A. (1990) The work of the National Health Service Central Register, *Population Trends*, 62: 29–32.

Frankel, S., Davison, C. and Davey Smith, G. (1991) Lay epidemiology and the rationality of responses to health education, *British Journal of General Practice*, 41: 428–30.

Frankenberg, R. (1994) The impact of HIV/AIDS on concepts relating to risk and culture within British community epidemiology: candidates or targets for prevention, *Social Science and Medicine*, 38: 1325–35.

Gardner, M., Hall, A., Downs, S. and Terrell, J. (1987a) Follow-up study of children born elsewhere but attending schools in Seascale, West Cumbria (schools cohort), *British Medical Journal*, 295: 819–22.

Gardner, M., Hall, A., Downs, S. and Terrell, J. (1987b) Follow-up study of children born to mothers resident in Seascale, West Cumbria (birth cohort), *British Medical Journal*, 295: 822–7.

Gardner, M., Snee, M., Hall, A., Powell, C., Downs, S. and Terrell, J. (1990a) Results of case-control study of leukaemia and lymphoma among young people near the Sellafield nuclear plant in West Cumbria, *British Medical Journal*, 300: 423–9.

Gardner, M., Hall, A., Snee, M., Downs, S., Powell, C. and Terrell, J. (1990b) Methods and basic data of case-control study of leukaemia and lymphoma among young people near the Sellafield nuclear plant in West Cumbria, *British Medical Journal*, 300: 429–34.

Giddens, A. (1991) *Modernity and Self-identity: Self and Society in the Late Modern Age*. Cambridge: Polity Press.

Gifford, S. (1986) The meaning of lumps: a case study in the ambiguities of risk, in C. Janes, R. Stall and S. Gifford (eds) *Anthropology and Epidemiology: Interdisciplinary Approaches to the Study of Health and Disease*. Dordrecht: Reidel.

Glanville, J., Haines, M. and Auston, I. (1998) Finding information on clinical effectiveness, *British Medical Journal*, 317: 72–6.

Gordis, L. (1996) *Epidemiology*. Pennsylvania: Saunders.

Gould, M. (1992) The use of GIS and CAC by Health Authorities: results from a postal questionnaire, *Area*, 24: 391–401.

Gould M. and Jones K. (1996) Analysing perceived limiting long-term illness using UK Census Microdata, *Social Science and Medicine*, 42: 857–69.

Government Statistical Service (1995) *Ordinary and Day Case Admissions: Financial Year 1994–95*. London: Department of Health.

Government Statistical Service (1996a) *Hospital Episode Statistics: Finished Consultant Episodes: Administration Statistics, England Financial Year 1994/95*. London: Department of Health.

Government Statistical Service (1996b) *Hospital Episode Statistics: Finished Consultant Episodes by Diagnosis and Operative Procedure: Injury/Poisoning by External Cause, England Financial Year 1994/95*. London: Department of Health.

Government Statistical Service (1996c) *Hospital Episode Statistics: Finished Consultant Episodes: Waiting Times, England Financial Year 1994/95*. London: Department of Health.

Graham, H. (1987) Women's smoking and family health, *Social Science and Medicine*, 25: 47–56.

Greenhalgh, T. (1997) *How to Read a Paper: The Basics of Evidence Based Medicine*. London: BMJ Publishing Group.

Greenhalgh, T. and Taylor, R. (1997) How to read a paper: papers that go beyond numbers (qualitative research), *British Medical Journal*, 315: 740–3.

Grol, R. (1997) Beliefs and evidence in changing clinical practice, *British Medical Journal*, 315: 418–21.

Guyatt, G. and Rennie, D. (1993) Users' guides to the medical literature, *Journal of the American Medical Association*, 270: 2096–7.

Guyatt, G.H., Sackett, D.L. and Cook, D.J. (1993) Users' guides to the medical literature, II: How to use an article about therapy or prevention: A. Are the results of the study valid? *Journal of the American Medical Association*, 270: 2598–601.

Guyatt, G.H., Sackett, D.L. and Cook, D.J. (1994) Users' guides to the medical literature, II: How to use an article about therapy or prevention: B. What were the results and will they help me in caring for my patients? *Journal of the American Medical Association*, 271: 59–63.

Harrison, G., Mason, P., Glazebrook, C., Medley, I., Croudace, T. and Docherty, S. (1994) Residence of incident cohort of psychotic patients after 13 years of follow up, *British Medical Journal*, 308: 813–16.

Hattersley, L. and Creeser, R. (1995) *The Longitudinal Study 1971 to 1991: History, Organisation and Quality of Data*, OPCS series LS No. 7. London: HMSO.

Herzlich, C. and Pierret, J. (1987) *Illness and Self in Society*. Baltimore: Johns Hopkins University Press.

Hill, A. (1965) The environment and disease: association and causation, *Proceedings of the Royal Society of Medicine*, 58: 295–300.

Hoinville, G., Jowell, R. and Airey, C. (1977) *Survey Research Practice*. London: Heinemann.

Jackson, P. (1994) Passive smoking and ill-health: practice and process in the production of medical knowledge, *Sociology of Health and Illness*, 16: 423–47.

Jarman, B. (1983) Identification of underprivileged areas, *British Medical Journal*, 286: 1705–9.

Jarman, B. (1984) Underprivileged areas: validation and distribution of scores, *British Medical Journal*, 289: 1587–92.

Jones, K. and Moon, G. (1987) *Health, Disease and Society*. London: Routledge.

Jones, K., Moon, G. and Clegg, A. (1991) Ecological and individual effects in childhood immunisation uptake: a multi-level approach, *Social Science and Medicine*, 33: 501–8.

Joseph, A. and Phillips, D. (1984) *Accessibility and Utilization: Geographical Perspectives on Health*. London: Harper & Row.

Kinnear, P. and Gray, C. (1997) *SPSS for Windows Made Simple*. Hove: Psychology Press.

Kirkwood, B. (1988) *Essentials of Medical Statistics*. Blackwell: Oxford.

Kivell, P., Turton, B. and Dawson, B. (1990) Neighbourhoods for health service administration, *Social Science and Medicine*, 30: 701–11.

Koepsell, T. (1998a) Community trials, in P. Armitage and T. Colton (eds) *Encyclopedia of Biostatistics*. Chichester: John Wiley.

Koepsell, T. (1998b) Community trials, in R. Brownson and D. Petitti (eds) *Applied Epidemiology*. Oxford: Open University Press.

Krieger, N. and Birn, A. (1998) A vision of social justice as the foundation of public health: commemorating 150 years of the spirit of 1848, *American Journal of Public Health*, 88: 1603–6.

Krieger, N., Rowley, D., Herman, A., Avery, B. and Phillips, M. (1993) Racism, sexism and social class: implications for studies of health, disease, and well-being, *American Journal of Preventive Medicine*, 9 (Supplement): 82–112.

Langham, S., Normand, C., Piercy, J. and Rose, G. (1994) Coronary heart disease, in A. Stevens and J. Raftery (eds) *Health Care Needs Assessment*. Oxford: Radcliffe Medical Press.

Leck, I. (1989) The north–south divide in England: implications for health care resource allocation, *Community Medicine*, 11: 102–7.

Li Wan Po, A. (1998) *Dictionary of Evidence-based Medicine*. Edinburgh: Churchill Livingstone.

Lilienfeld, A. and Lilienfeld, D. (1980) *Foundations of Epidemiology*. Oxford: Oxford University Press.

Litva, A. and Eyles, J. (1994) Health or healthy: why people are not sick in a southern Ontario town, *Social Science and Medicine*, 39: 1083–91.

Loomis, D. and Wing, S. (1991) Is molecular epidemiology a germ theory for the end of the twentieth century? *International Journal of Epidemiology*, 19: 1–3.

Lupton, D. (1995) *The Imperative of Health: Public Health and the Regulated Body*. London: Sage.

Lupton, D. (1996) *Food, the Body and the Self*. London: Sage.

Lupton, D. (1997) *Medicine as Culture*. London: Sage.

MacMahon, B. and Pugh, T. (1970) *Epidemiologic Methods*. Boston: Little Brown.

Mantel, N. and Haenszel, W. (1959) Statistical aspects of the analysis of data from retrospective studies of disease, *Journal of the National Cancer Institute*, 22: 719–48.

Marmot, M. and Brunner, E. (1991) Alcohol and cardiovascular disease: the status of the U shaped curve, *British Medical Journal*, 303: 565–8.

Marsh, C. (1988) *Exploring Data*. Cambridge: Polity Press.

Marsh, C. (1993a) The validation of census data, in A. Dale and C. Marsh (eds) *The 1991 Census Users' Guide*. London: HMSO.

Marsh, C. (1993b) The sample of anonymised records, in A. Dale and C. Marsh (eds) *The 1991 Census Users' Guide*. London: HMSO.

Martin, D. (1991) *Geographic Information Systems and their Socioeconomic Applications*. London: Routledge.

Martin, D. (1995) Censuses and the modelling of population in GIS, in P. Longley and G. Clarke (eds) *GIS for Business and Service Planning*. Cambridge: GeoInformation International.

Martin, D., Harris, J., Sadler, J. and Tate, N. (1998) Putting the Census on the web: lessons from two case studies, *Area*, 30: 311–20.

McKinlay, J. (1993) The promotion of health through planned sociopolitical change: challenges for research and policy, *Social Science and Medicine*, 36: 109–17.

McKinlay, J. (1996) Some contributions from the social system to gender inequalities in heart disease, *Journal of Health and Social Behaviour*, 37: 1–26.

McNeil, D. (1996) *Epidemiological Research Methods*. Chichester: John Wiley.

Medical Research Council (1948) Streptomycin treatment in pulmonary tuberculosis, *British Medical Journal*, ii: 769.

Mellin, G. and Katzenstein, M. (1962) The saga of thalidomide: neutrophy to embyopathy, with case reports of congenital anomalies, *New England Journal of Medicine*, 267: 1184–93, 1238–43.

Mile, R. and Chambers, L. (1993) Assessing the scientific quality of review articles, *Journal of Epidemiology and Community Health*, 47: *169–70.*

Mohan, J. (1995) *A National Health Service? The Restructuring of Health Care in Britain Since 1979.* Basingstoke: Macmillan.

Mohan, J., Johnson, K., Chambers, J., McKenzie, J. and Killoran, A. (1990) *Mapping the Epidemic: Coronary Heart Disease.* London: Health Education Authority.

Moon, G., Iggulden, P. and Neira-Muñoz, E. (1998) Resource allocation for primary psychiatric care: a fine-scale, needs-based approach, in *Géographie et Socio-économie de la Santé: Allocation des Ressources, Géographie des Soins.* Paris: CREDES.

More, A. and Martin, D. (1998) Quantitative health research in an emerging information economy, *Health and Place*, 4: 213–22.

Morris, J. (1975) *The Uses of Epidemiology.* Oxford: Churchill Livingstone.

Morris, J. (chair) (1968) Controlled trial of soya bean oil and myocardial infarction, *The Lancet*, 2: 693.

Moser, C. and Kalton, G. (1971) *Survey Methods in Social Investigation.* Aldershot: Dartmouth.

Mould, R. (1983) *Cancer Statistics.* Bristol: Adam Hilger.

Muir Gray, J. (1997) *Evidence-based Healthcare: How to Make Health Policy and Management Decisions.* Edinburgh: Churchill Livingstone.

Mundell, I. (1993) Peering through the smoke screen, *New Scientist*, 9: 14–15.

NHSE (NHS Executive) (1996a) Burdens of Disease: A Discussion Document. Leeds: NHS Executive.

NHSE (NHS Executive) (1996b) *Information on Clinical Effectiveness.* Leeds: NHS Executive.

ONS (1996) *Key Health Statistics from General Practice.* London: The Stationery Office.

ONS (1997a) *English Life Tables*, series DS No. 15. London: The Stationery Office.

ONS (1997b) *The Health of Adult Britain 1841–1994.* London: The Stationery Office.

ONS (1998) *Living in Britain: Results from the 1996 General Household Survey.* London: The Stationery Office.

OPCS (Office of Population Censuses and Surveys) (1990) *Mortality and Geography: Commentary*, series DS No. 9. London: HMSO.

OPCS (Office of Population Censuses and Surveys) (1992a) *Making a Population Estimate in England and Wales*, OPCS Occasional Paper No. 37. London: HMSO.

OPCS (Office of Population Censuses and Surveys) (1992b) *Provisional Mid-1991 Population Estimates in England and Wales and Constituent Local and Health Authorities based on 1991 Census Results*, OPCS Monitor 1, 92/1. London: HMSO.

OPCS (Office of Population Censuses and Surveys) (1995*) Morbidity Statistics from General Practice Fourth National Study 1991–1992*, series MB5 No. 3. London: HMSO.

OPCS (Office of Population Censuses and Surveys) (n.d.) *Area Mortality 1979–83*, Decennial Supplement Microfiche Tables. London: HMSO.

OPCS/RGO(S) (Office of Population Censuses and Surveys/Registrar General's Office (Scotland)) (1991) *Topic Statistics: Limiting Long-term Illness*, Census Guide No. 5. Fareham: OPCS.

Openshaw, S., Craft, A., Charlton, M. and Birch, J. (1988) Investigation of leukae-
    mia clusters by use of a geographical analysis machine, *The Lancet*, 6 February,
    272–3.
Oxman, A.D., Cook, D.J. and Guyatt, G.H. (1994) Users' guides to the medical
    literature, VI: How to use an overview, *Journal of the American Medical Association*,
    272: 1367–71.
Pearce, N. (1996) Traditional epidemiology, modern epidemiology, and public health,
    American Journal of Public Health, 86: 678–83.
Pearce, N., Prior, I., Methven, D. *et al.* (1990) Follow-up of New Zealand partici-
    pants in British atmospheric nuclear weapons tests in the Pacific, *British Medical
    Journal*, 300: 1161–6.
Peele, S. (1993) The conflict between public health goals and the temperance men-
    tality, *American Journal of Public Health*, 18: 805–10.
Peterson, A. and Lupton, D. (1996) *The New Public Health: Health and Self in the Age
    of Risk*. London: Sage.
Pill, R. and Stott, N. (1982) Concepts of illness causation and responsibility: some
    preliminary data from a sample of working class mothers, *Social Science and
    Medicine*, 16: 43–52.
Pocock, S. (1983) *Clinical Trials: A Practical Approach*. Chichester: John Wiley.
Pollock, K. (1988) On the nature of social stress: the production of modern mytho-
    logy, *Social Science and Medicine*, 26(3): 381–92.
Popay, J. and Williams, G. (1996) Public health research and lay knowledge, *Social
    Science and Medicine*, 42: 759–68.
Portsmouth and South East Hampshire Health Authority (1990) *Community Health
    Atlas*. Portsmouth: Portsmouth and South East Hampshire Health Authority.
Portsmouth and South East Hampshire Health Authority (1996) *Community Health
    Atlas*, 4th edition. Portsmouth: Portsmouth and SE Hampshire Health Authority.
Potter, J., Wetherell, M. and Chitty, A. (1991) Quantification rhetoric: cancer on
    television, *Discourse and Society*, 2: 33–65.
Prescott-Clarke, P. and Primatesta, P. (eds) (1996) *Health Survey for England 1994*.
    London: The Stationery Office.
Prior, L. (1985) The social production of mortality statistics, *Sociology of Health and
    Illness*, 7: 220–35.
Prior, L. and Bloor, M. (1993) Why people die: social representations of death and
    its causes, *Science as Culture*, 3: 346–75.
Puska, P. (1990) *Comprehensive Cardiovascular Community Control Programmes in
    Europe*. Copenhagen: WHO Regional Office for Europe.
Rees, P. (1994) Estimating and projecting the populations of urban communities,
    Environment and Planning A, 26: 1671–97.
Rhind, D. (1983) Creating new variables and new areas from the census data, in
    D. Rhind (ed.) *A Census User's Handbook*. London: Methuen.
Roht, L. (1982) *Principles of Epidemiology*. New York: Academic Press.
Rose, D., Buck, N. and Johnston, R. (1994) The British Household Panel Study: a
    valuable new resource for geographical research, *Area*, 26: 368–76.
Rose, G. and Barker, D. (1986) *Epidemiology for the Uninitiated*, 2nd edition. London:
    BMJ Publishing Group.
Rose, G., McCartney, P. and Reid, D. (1977) Self administration of a questionnaire
    on chest pain and intermittent claudication, *British Journal of Preventative and
    Social Medicine*, 31: 42–8.
Rose, N. and Miller, P. (1992) Political power beyond the state: problematics of
    government, *British Journal of Sociology*, 43: 173–205.
Sackett, D. Haynes, R. and Tugwell, P. (eds) (1991) *Clinical Epidemiology: A Basic
    Science For Clinical Medicine*, 2nd edition. Boston: Little Brown.
Sackett, D., Richardson, W., Rosenburg, W. and Haynes, R. (1997) *Evidence-based
    Medicine: How to Practise and Teach EBM*. Edinburgh: Churchill Livingstone.

Salisbury, D. and Begg, N. (eds) (1996) *Immunisation Against Infectious Diseases*, 2nd edition. London: HMSO.

Sanderson, H., Anthony, P. and Mountney, L. (eds) (1998) *Casemix for All*. Oxford: Radcliffe Medical Press.

Sayer, A. (1992) *Method in Social Science: A Realist Approach*. London: Routledge.

Schiller, N., Crystal, S. and Llewellen, D. (1994) Risky business: the cultural construction of AIDS risk groups, *Social Science and Medicine*, 38: 1337–46.

Schwab, M. and Syme, S. (1997) On paradigms, community participation, and the future of public health, *American Journal of Public Health*, 87: 2049–52.

Scott-Samuel, A. (1981) Towards a socialist epidemiology, *Radical Community Medicine*, 7 (Summer): 13–18.

Senior, M. (1991) Deprivation payments to GPs: not what the doctor ordered, *Environment and Planning, C: Government and Policy*, 9: 79–84.

Shaper, A., Cook, D., Walker, M. and MacFarlane, P. (1984) Prevalence of ischaemic heart disease in middle aged British men, *British Heart Journal*, 51: 595–605.

Silagy, C., Mant, D., Fowler, G. and Lodge, M. (1994) Meta-analysis on efficacy of nicotine replacement therapies in smoking cessation, *The Lancet*, 343: 139–42.

Simpson, S. (ed.) (1998) *Making Local Population Statistics: A Guide for Practitioners*. Wokingham: Local Authorities Research and Intelligence Association.

Simpson, S., Middleton, L., Diamond, I. and Lunn, D. (1997) Small-area population estimates: a review of methods used in Britain in the 1990s, *International Journal of Population Geography*, 3: 265–80.

Smith, B. (1981) Black lung: the social production of disease, *International Journal of Health Services*, 11: 343–59.

Snow, J. ([1855] 1936) *On the Mode of Communication of Cholera*. Boston: Harvard University Press.

SSRU (Social Statistics Research Unit) (1990) OPCS *Longitudinal Study User Manual*. London: SSRU, City University.

Staus, S. and Sackett, D. (1998) Using research findings in clinical practice, *British Medical Journal*, 317: 339–42.

Sterling, T. (1978) Does smoking kill workers or working kill smokers? Or the mutual relationship between smoking, occupation and respiratory disease, *International Journal of Health Services*, 8: 437–52.

Sterling, T. and Weinkam, J. (1990) The confounding of occupation and smoking and its consequences, *Social Science and Medicine*, 30: 457–67.

Stevens, A. and Raftery, J. (eds) (1994) *Health Care Needs Assessment: The Epidemiologically Based Needs Assessment Reviews*. Oxford: Radcliffe Medical Press.

Syme, S. (1996) To prevent disease: the need for a new approach, in D. Blane, E. Brunner and R. Wilkinson (eds) *Health and Social Organization: Towards a Health Policy for the 21st Century*. London: Routledge.

Thomas, J. (1998) Coronary artery disease in women: a historical perspective, *Archives of Internal Medicine*, 158: 333–7.

Townsend, P., Phillimore, P. and Beatie, A. (1988) *Health and Deprivation: Inequality and the North*. London: Croom Helm.

Treichler, P. (1988) AIDS, gender, and biomedical discourse: current contexts for meaning, in E. Fee and D. Fox. (eds) *AIDS: Burdens of History*. Berkeley: University of California Press.

Treichler, P. (1992) AIDS, HIV, and the cultural construction of reality, in G. Herdt and S. Lindenbaum (eds) *The Time of AIDS: Social Analysis, Theory, and Method*. London: Sage.

Turner, B. (1992) *Regulating Bodies: Essays in Medical Sociology*. London: Routledge.

Twigg, L. (1990) Health based geographical information systems: their potential examined in the light of existing data source, *Social Science and Medicine*, 30: 143–55.

Twigg, L. (1999) Choosing a national survey to investigate smoking behaviour: making comparisons between the General Household Survey, the British Household Panel Survey and the Health Survey for England, *Journal of Public Health Medicine*, 21: 14–21.

Twigg, L., Moon, G. and Jones, K. (2000) Predicting small-area health-related behaviour: a comparison of smoking and drinking indicators, *Social Science and Medicine*, 50: 1109–20.

Unwin, N., Carr, S. and Leeson, J. with Pless-Mulloli, T. (1997) *An Introductory Study Guide to Public Health and Epidemiology*. Buckingham: Open University Press.

Wakeford, R. (1998) Epidemiology and litigation – the Sellafield childhood leukaemia cases, *Journal of the Royal Statistical Society Series A*, 161: 313–25.

Wallace, M. and Denham, C. (1996) *The ONS Classification of Local and Health Authorities of Great Britain*, Studies on Medical and Population Subjects No. 59. London: HMSO.

Wenger, N. (1997) Coronary heart disease: an older woman's major health risk, *British Medical Journal*, 315: 1085–90.

WHO (World Health Organization) (1995) Annual Report. Geneva: WHO.

Wiggins, R. (1993) The validation of census data. I: post-enumeration survey approaches, in A. Dale and C. Marsh (eds) *The 1991 Census Users' Guide*. London: HMSO.

Wild, S. and McKeigue, P. (1997) Cross-sectional analysis of mortality by country of birth in England and Wales, 1970–92, *British Medical Journal*, 314: 705.

Wiles, R. (1998) Patients' perception of their heart attack and recovery: the influence of epidemiological 'evidence' and personal experience, *Social Science and Medicine*, 46: 1477–86.

Williams, R. (1983) Concepts of health: an analysis of lay logic, *Sociology*, 17: 185–205.

Wing, S. (1994) The limits of epidemiology, *Medicine and Global Survival*, 1: 74–86.

Wright, P. (1988) Babyhood: the social construction of infant care as a medical problem in England in the years around 1900, in M. Lock and D. Gordon (eds) *Biomedicine Examined*. Dordrecht: Kluwer.

Wrigley, N. (1991) Market-based systems of health-care provision, the NHS Bill, and geographical information systems, *Environment and Planning A*, 23: 5–8.

Zierler, S. and Krieger, N. (1998) HIV infection in women: social inequalities as determinants of risk, *Critical Public Health*, 8: 13–32.

INDEX

COMMUNITY CARE FOR NURSES AND THE CARING PROFESSIONS

Nigel Malin, Jill Manthorpe, David Race and Stephen Wilmot

This textbook provides a concise introduction to policy and practice issues in community care. It has been written for nurses and other health professionals in training, particularly those wishing to specialize in community care. It explains the concepts behind community care policy and demonstrates their relevance to work in healthcare settings.

In a clear, accessible way, the authors draw together a wide range of material on the changing nature of community care, assess current research evidence and examine the central issues relating to everyday practice. Each chapter has a similar structure, with an introductory and concluding section making it ideal for use as a teaching text. At the end of each chapter there are suggestions for further reading and follow-up work. Students will also find key points and concepts listed throughout the text which are explained in a helpful glossary at the end of the book.

Contents

The policy context – Background developments, 1957–88 – The reforms and the mixed economy – Towards a conceptual framework – Values, assumptions and ideologies – Values, theories and realities: The case of learning disability services – Users' and carers' perspectives – Users' perspectives: Do services empower users? – Carers' perspectives: Do services support carers? – Professional directions – Professions in community care – Teams in community care – Glossary – Index.

224pp   0 335 19670 5   (Paperback)   0 335 19671 3   (Hardback)

PSYCHOLOGY FOR NURSES AND THE CARING PROFESSIONS
Sheila Payne and Jan Walker

- What is psychology and how is it relevant to health care practice?
- What influences do psychological factors have in determining outcomes in health care?
- What are the different approaches within psychology which can be used to understand normal human functioning?

Psychology for Nurses and the Caring Professions is one of a series of texts which provide coherent and multi-disciplinary support for all professional groups involved in the provision of health and social care. It introduces students to a range of psychological theories and research, supported by evidence from health psychology. Applications are offered within a variety of health care settings, with an emphasis on health promotion and preventive care.

The authors draw upon their clinical, teaching and research experience to engage the student's interest through the use of case examples, special research-based topics and exercises for group discussion or individual study. The text has been carefully designed with the student in mind: a comprehensive reference list is provided at the end of the book, together with a glossary of terms. The text is illustrated throughout with diagrams, tables and graphs and suggestions for further reading are given at the end of each chapter.

Psychology for Nurses and the Caring Professions is a key textbook for all students undertaking diploma or degree level courses in nursing, health and social care.

Contents
Introduction to psychology – Understanding health and illness – Self concept and body image – Theories of learning developments and applications – Perception, memory and patient information-giving – Stress and coping: theory and applications in health care – Development and loss in social relationships – Pain – Social processes in health care delivery – Epilogue – Glossary – References – Index.

240pp   0 335 19410 9   (Paperback)   0 335 19411 7   (Hardback)

RESEARCH INTO PRACTICE (SECOND EDITION)
A READER FOR NURSES AND THE CARING PROFESSIONS

Pamela Abbott and Roger Sapsford (eds)

Praise for the first edition of *Research into Practice* and *Research Methods for Nurses and the Caring Professions*:

> These books provide a good introduction for the uninitiated to reading and doing research. Abbott and Sapsford provide a clearly written and accessible introduction to social research . . . One of their aims is to 'de-mystify' research, and in this they succeed admirably . . . After reading the text and the articles in the reader, and working through the various research exercises, readers should have a clear appreciation of how to evaluate other people's research and how to begin their own.
>
> David Field, Journal of Palliative Medicine

This is a thoroughly revised and updated edition of the bestselling reader for nurses and the caring professions. It offers carefully selected examples of research, all concerned in some way with nursing or the study of health and community care. It illustrates the kind of research that can be done by a small team or a single researcher, without large-scale research grants. The editors have chosen papers which show a great diversity of approaches: differing in emphasis on description or explanation, different degrees of structure in design and different appeals to the authority of science or the authenticity of emphatic exploration. They show the limitations typical of small-scale projects carried out with limited resources and the experience of applied research as it occurs in practice, as opposed to how it tends to look when discussed in textbooks. The chapters have been organized into three sections representing three distinct types of social science research: observing and participating, talking to people and asking questions, and controlled trials and comparisons. Each section is provided with an editorial introduction.

Contents
Introduction – Section A: Observing and participating – Labouring in the dark: limitations on the giving of information to enable patients to orient themselves to the likely events and timescale of labour – Portfolios: a developmental influence? – A postscript to nursing – Section B: Talking to people and asking questions – Leaving it to mum: community care for mentally handicapped children – Planning research: a case of heart disease – Home helps and district nurses: community care in the far South-west – Studying policy and practice: use of vignettes – Section C: Controlled trials and comparisons – Treatment of depressed women by nurses in Britain – The mortality of doctors in relation to their smoking habits: a preliminary report – Ethnic variation in the female labour force: a research note – Postscript – Author index – Subject index.

The Contributors
Pamela Abbott, Julia V. Cayne, Richard Doll, Verona Gordon, A. Bradford Hill, Nicky James, Mavis Kirkham, Roger Sapsford, Melissa Tyler.

184pp   0 335 19695 0   (Paperback)   0 335 19696 9   (Hardback)

RESEARCH METHODS FOR NURSES AND THE CARING PROFESSIONS (SECOND EDITION)

Pamela Abbott and Roger Sapsford

Praise for the first editions of *Research into Practice* and *Research Methods for Nurses and the Caring Professions*:

> These books provide a good introduction for the uninitiated to reading and doing research. Abbott and Sapsford provide a clearly written and accessible introduction to social research . . . One of their aims is to 'de-mystify' research, and in this they succeed admirably . . . After reading the text and the articles in the reader, and working through the various research exercises, readers should have a clear appreciation of how to evaluate other people's research and how to begin their own.
>
> David Field, *Journal of Palliative Medicine*

This book, now substantially revised in its second edition, is about the appreciation, evaluation and conduct of social research. Aimed at nurses, social workers, community workers and others in the caring professions, the book is particularly focused on research which evaluates and contributes to professional practice. The authors have provided many short, practical exercises in the text, and the examples are drawn mostly from projects carried out by one or two people rather than large research teams. The clear, accessible style will make this the ideal introductory text for those undertaking or studying research for the first time.

The book may be used in conjunction with *Research into Practice* (Open University Press), a reader of useful examples selected by the same authors.

Contents

224pp   0 335 19697 7   (Paperback)   0 335 19698 5   (Hardback)

SOCIAL PERSPECTIVES ON PREGNANCY AND CHILDBIRTH FOR MIDWIVES, NURSES AND THE CARING PROFESSIONS

Julie Kent

- How does pregnancy and childbirth affect women's lives?
- How do we understand the connections between the biological and social processes that shape experiences of pregnancy and childbirth?
- What influences contemporary approaches to maternity care and midwifery education?

This book explores contemporary issues around pregnancy and childbirth using a feminist sociological approach. Becoming pregnant and giving birth are seen here as complex social processes. The book therefore goes beyond biological accounts of pregnancy and childbirth to examine these social processes. The biological and the social are seen as linked together. Knowledge, power, identity and the body are key concepts in the book and important for understanding the relationship between the biological and social. Written in a clear, accessible style the text will assist nurses, midwives and the caring professions to use sociological ideas and theories. It is divided into four parts that look at ways of knowing, the professionals, constructing identities and women's bodies. In the conclusion the author discusses the implications of adopting a feminist and sociological approach to health care practice.

Social Perspectives on Pregnancy and Childbirth has been designed for use as a key text on a range of pre-registration and post-registration degree courses for nurses and midwives, and is suitable for use on a range of undergraduate programmes in social science and health studies.

Contents
Part 1: The biological and the social – Who knows best? Competing approaches to childbirth – Part 2: The professionals – Educating the professionals – Midwifery as 'women's work' – Part 3: Constructing identities – Women as mothers – Sexual identities – Part 4: Women's bodies – Reproductive technologies and the new genetics – Imagining bodies – Changing childbirth, changing the future? – References – Index.

272pp   0 335 19911 9   (Paperback)   0 335 19912 7   (Hardback)

SOCIAL POLICY FOR NURSES AND THE CARING PROFESSIONS

Louise Ackers and Pamela Abbott

- What is the relationship between social policy and health?
- Who provides social welfare?
- How has the provision of welfare developed?

Social Policy for Nurses and the Caring Professions is one of a series of texts which provide coherent and multi-disciplinary support for all professional groups involved in the provision of health and social care. It provides the student with a lively, readable and well illustrated introduction to social policy. The authors take as a starting point the importance of the conceptual connection between health and illness. The stress throughout the book is on the significance of social policy in preventing ill health and disability as well as supporting the sick and disabled. A broad approach to social policy is taken, and the text is organized around the provision of welfare in the following contexts:

- public
- private
- voluntary
- informal.

Consideration is given to competing ideologies of welfare and the development of welfare as well as contemporary provision.

Social Policy for Nurses and the Caring Professions is based on the authors' first-hand teaching and research experience. The text has been carefully designed with the student in mind: a comprehensive reference list is provided at the end of the book, together with a glossary of important terms. The text is illustrated with tables and graphs throughout, and there are suggestions for further reading at the end of each chapter.

Social Policy for Nurses and the Caring Professions is a key textbook for all students undertaking diploma or degree level courses in nursing, health and social care.

Contents

What is social policy? – The development of a welfare state – Health inequalities and state health policies – Poverty, inequality and social policy – State income maintenance and welfare benefits – Privatization and social welfare – The changing role of the voluntary sector in the provision of social welfare – The role of informal care – The mixed economy of care: welfare services for dependent people – Welfare pluralism in the 1990s: the changing role of the state – Glossary – References – Index.

288pp   0 335 19359 5   (Paperback)   0 335 19360 9   (Hardback)